1,000,000 Books
are available to read at

Forgotten Books

www.ForgottenBooks.com

Read online
Download PDF
Purchase in print

ISBN 978-0-260-23867-2
PIBN 11012641

This book is a reproduction of an important historical work. Forgotten Books uses
state-of-the-art technology to digitally reconstruct the work, preserving the original format
whilst repairing imperfections present in the aged copy. In rare cases, an imperfection in
the original, such as a blemish or missing page, may be replicated in our edition. We do,
however, repair the vast majority of imperfections successfully; any imperfections that
remain are intentionally left to preserve the state of such historical works.

Forgotten Books is a registered trademark of FB &c Ltd.
Copyright © 2018 FB &c Ltd.
FB &c Ltd, Dalton House, 60 Windsor Avenue, London, SW19 2RR.
Company number 08720141. Registered in England and Wales.

For support please visit www.forgottenbooks.com

1 MONTH OF FREE READING

at

www.ForgottenBooks.com

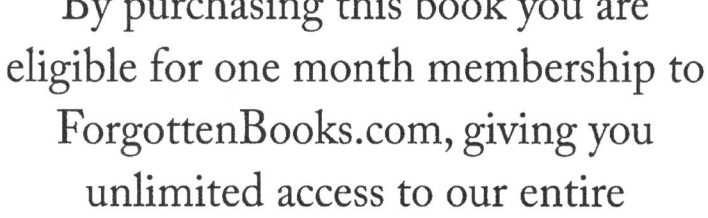

By purchasing this book you are eligible for one month membership to ForgottenBooks.com, giving you unlimited access to our entire collection of over 1,000,000 titles via our web site and mobile apps.

To claim your free month visit:
www.forgottenbooks.com/free1012641

* Offer is valid for 45 days from date of purchase. Terms and conditions apply.

English
Français
Deutsche
Italiano
Español
Português

www.forgottenbooks.com

Mythology Photography **Fiction** Fishing Christianity **Art** Cooking Essays Buddhism Freemasonry Medicine **Biology** Music **Ancient Egypt** Evolution Carpentry Physics Dance Geology **Mathematics** Fitness Shakespeare **Folklore** Yoga Marketing **Confidence** Immortality Biographies Poetry **Psychology** Witchcraft Electronics Chemistry History **Law** Accounting **Philosophy** Anthropology Alchemy Drama Quantum Mechanics Atheism Sexual Health **Ancient History Entrepreneurship** Languages Sport Paleontology Needlework Islam **Metaphysics** Investment Archaeology Parenting Statistics Criminology **Motivational**

PRACTICAL
OBSERVATIONS
ON THE
SYMPTOMS, DISCRIMINATION, AND TREATMENT,

OF SOME OF THE MOST IMPORTANT

DISEASES

OF THE

LOWER INTESTINES AND ANUS.

PARTICULARLY INCLUDING

THOSE AFFECTIONS PRODUCED BY STRICTURE, ULCERATION, AND TUMOUR, WITHIN THE CAVITY OF THE RECTUM, AND PILES, FISTULÆ, AND EXCRESCENCES, FORMED AT ITS EXTERNAL OPENING.

ILLUSTRATED BY NUMEROUS CASES.

To which are added,

SOME SUGGESTIONS UPON A NEW AND SUCCESSFUL MODE OF CORRECTING HABITUAL CONFINEMENT IN THE BOWELS, TO ENSURE THEIR REGULAR ACTION WITHOUT THE AID OF PURGATIVES; ON A PRINCIPLE ESSENTIALLY CONDUCIVE TO THE PREVENTION OF THE ABOVE DISEASES.

By JOHN HOWSHIP,

Member of the Royal College of Surgeons, in London; of the Société Médicale D'Emulation, in Paris, and of the Medico-Chirurgical Society, London: Author of Practical Observations in Surgery, and Morbid Anatomy; and of Practical Observations on the Diseases of the Urinary Organs.

FIRST AMERICAN FROM THE SECOND LONDON EDITION.

PHILADELPHIA:
PUBLISHED BY BENJAMIN WARNER, AND SOLD ALSO AT HIS STORES IN RICHMOND, VA. AND LOUISVILLE, KEN.
AND BY
W. P. BASON, CHARLESTON, S. C.

1821.
FRANKISH, PRINTER.

WIB
H866p
1821a

TO
ROBERT HOOPER, M.D. F.L.S.

BACHELOR OF PHYSIC, OF THE UNIVERSITY OF OXFORD;
MEMBER OF THE ROYAL COLLEGE OF PHYSICIANS;
PHYSICIAN TO THE MARYLEBONE INFIRMARY;
&c. &c. &c.

My dear Sir,

As one of my earliest professional friends, and as one of the most highly respected of my professional teachers, I took the liberty of dedicating the first edition of this work to you; with a candid acknowledgment of my being induced so to do, by the conviction, that from you this essay would be sure to obtain full credit for any value it might possess, and that through your distinguished name and patronage it would be also sure of finding a more favourable reception with the public.

That these expectations have not been altogether disappointed, I may perhaps, venture to believe, from the interval of a few months only having elapsed between the publication of the first, and the necessity for printing the second impression; which impression I trust you will find I have taken some pains to render more worthy of your approbation, and at the same time, more generally useful to the profession.

With every sentiment of respect
and gratitude,
Believe me to remain,
Dear Sir,
Ever yours faithfully,
JOHN HOWSHIP.

Great George Street, Hanover Square.
Jan. 10. 1821.

CONTENTS

Introduction

CHAPTER I.

ON COMPARISON OF CHARACTERS IN THE SEXES

Part 1.

On the Colors of the Skin

Part 2.

On the Stiffness and Appearance

Part 3.

On the Treatment

CHAPTER II.

ON CAUSATION OF THE EXTERNAL APPEARED OF THE

Part 1.

On the Cause of the Disease

CONTENTS.

Introduction — Page ix

CHAPTER I.

ON CONTRACTION, OR STRICTURE IN THE RECTUM.

Sect. 1.

On the Causes of the Disease -

Sect. 2.

On the Symptoms and Appearances — 5

Sect. 3.

On the Treatment - - - - 16

CHAPTER II.

ON ULCERATION OF THE INTERNAL SURFACE OF THE INTESTINE.

Sect. 1.

On the Causes of the Disease - - 76

	Page
Sect. 2.	
On the Symptoms and Appearances -	80
Sect. 3.	
On the Treatment - - - -	90

CHAPTER III.

ON THE GROWTH OF TUMOURS WITHIN THE BOWEL.

Sect. 1.	
On the Causes of the Disease - -	118
Sect. 2.	
On the Symptoms and Appearances -	120
Sect. 3.	
On the Treatment - - - -	123

CHAPTER IV.

ON THE PROLAPSUS ANI, OR THE DESCENT OF THE BOWEL.

Sect. 1.	
On the Causes of the Disease - -	128
Sect. 2.	
On the Symptoms and Appearances -	129
Sect. 3.	
On the Treatment - - -	136

CHAPTER V.

ON HÆMORRHOIDAL TUMOURS, OR PILES.

Sect. 1.

On the Causes of the Disease — — 169

Sect. 2.

On the Symptoms and Appearances — 170

Sect. 3.

On the Treatment — — — — 176

CHAPTER VI.

ON FISTULA IN ANO.

Sect. 1.

On the Causes of the Disease — — 203

Sect. 2.

On the Symptoms and Appearances — 204

Sect. 3.

On the Treatment — — — — 208

CHAPTER VII.

ON THE HÆMORRHOIDAL EXCRESCENCE.

Sect. 1.

On the Causes of the Disease — — 222

Sect. 2.

On the Symptoms and Appearances — 223

SECT. 3.

On the Treatment - - - 226

CHAPTER VIII.

On the best Means for obtaining a Regular State and Action of the Bowels; as essentially conducive to the Prevention of the above Diseases. - - - - 228

INTRODUCTION.

The peculiar spirit of active research, that has distinguished many of the first characters in the present day, affords ample testimony that the real friends of scientific pursuits are both zealous and numerous.

Not only is the detail of minute structure in human anatomy more clearly unfolded to us by the combined labours of various individuals; but we also see the wide field of comparative anatomy entered upon with an avidity, and its devious paths sought out and explored with a degree of industry, talent, and success, heretofore unknown.

Those who consider the healing art with that attention its importance demands, must also admire the brilliancy of illustration which has of late been shed upon the elementary principles of the animal machine; their laws of combination, the chemical changes connected with the functions of vitality, and above all, those deep researches by which the progressive, yet mysterious conversions that take place in the nutritious fluid, have been unveiled, the newly acquired properties of the chyle ascertained, together with the succeeding changes by which that fluid is eventually identified with the general volume of circulating blood.

Neither are the great acquisitions to medical

science in the present day confined to anatomy and physiology. The unexampled assiduity displayed in the researches connected with chemical philosophy has thrown much essentially useful light upon the most secret operations of the animal economy under the influence of diseases; developing, with other matters of high importance, the precise composition of the various kinds of urinary concretions, and demonstrating that there are modes by which the calculous diathesis may be changed and corrected.

Among these who in the present age have most eminently distinguished themselves by their labours in physiology and comparative anatomy, may be ranked the late Mr. HUNTER, Sir EVERARD HOME, and Mons. CUVIER, each of whom have established high claims to public regard upon almost innumerable occasions. Physiology and pathology are also indebted for many things to the judicious and persevering application of Mr. BRODIE, especially for those experiments by which the importance of the nervous influence is demonstrated as the regulator of secretion, and the preserver of animal heat. In chemical science Sir HUMPHRY DAVY, and as regards the elucidation of animal chemistry, Professor BRANDE, have shone forth with permanent lustre, tracing out the previously hidden resources and operations of nature, and displaying with admirable skill many of the silent and secret agencies appointed to superintend the performance of the living functions.

There are in fact a host of labourers in the vineyard; many of whom have conferred essential obligations upon society, no less by the animating influence of their example, than by the intrinsic value of their personal contributions.

The following observations relate to a very important branch of surgical practice. The principal reasons for bringing them forward are, on the one hand, my having devoted a considerable portion of time to the study of these complaints, and on the other having had considerable opportunities for seeing them; and perhaps I may also add, rather considerable success either in relieving or removing them.

The functions assigned to the alimentary canal are various and interesting. This canal may be represented as a very extended tube, in some parts larger, in others smaller; in a certain portion endowed with a power of digesting its contents; but through its whole extent capable of contraction.

This power of contraction is of so much importance as to be in fact indispensable; the continual necessity for it being shown in the changes produced by digestion, which is the process appointed for the selection of the useful, and rejection of the useless parts of the food.

In one of the most correct, and at the same time comprehensive, medical works of the present day, the intestinal canal is defined to be " the convoluted tube that extends from the stomach to the anus; receives the injected food, retains it a certain time; mixes with it the bile and pancreatic juice; propels the chyle into the lacteals, and covers the fæces with mucus."*

The contractile power of the intestines resides in what has been termed the muscular coat, which coat is lined internally by a mucous membrane, and externally by a fine smooth membrane, that completes the structure of the tube; and as each of these expansions or coats is gifted with peculiar functions in health, so is each subject to peculiar complaints when under the influence of disease.

In the natural state, the internal membrane of the bowels secretes a limpid fluid, which tends to regulate the due consistence of the mass of contents, and facilitate their transit; this membrane also answers a purpose of essential importance in the economy, by absorbing or taking up the nutritive particles from the digested matter, which thence passes by the lacteal vessels into the general volume of the circulating blood.

In disease, this membrane is subject to all the effects of inflammation, particularly ulceration.

In the natural state, the circular fibres of the muscular coat of the bowels have the power of lessening the diameter of the intestine, and the longitudinal fibres of diminishing the length of any part of the canal; but in health these actions are altogether transitory and progressive, no portion of the tube ever remaining contracted, or dilated, permanently. Under disease, however, it is otherwise; from the influence of irritation any part of the canal may be subjected to spasm,

* Hooper's Medical Dictionary, 4th edition, 1820.

and should this connect itself with inflammation, the effusion of new matter may lay the foundation for some permanent disease.

The natural state of the external coat of the intestines, is that of a fine smooth and transparent membrane, which like most of the other textures in the body, is ultimately cellular, highly elastic, and moistened by a secretion of limpid fluid. From inflammation and other causes this membrane also is liable to become thickened, and otherwise diseased.

The following observations relate to the discrimination and management of those diseases to which the inferior parts of the alimentary canal are more particularly subject; diseases which are all of them important, all more or less distressing, some of them extremely painful, and many of them, if misunderstood or neglected, eventually fatal.

Almost every deviation from health, either in the functions or structure of the bowels, may be considered as connected with one of two states, for almost every case will manifest either excess, or deficiency, in tone, or power of action; the first state favouring the production of inflammation, contraction, or stricture, ulceration, abscess, and fistulæ; the second inducing hæmorrhoidal tumours, hæmorrhages, and prolapsus.

In no department of surgery is the safety of the patient more immediately concerned, or the discernment of the practitioner more promptly required, than in ascertaining the early approach of some of these complaints; and no adequate series of observations upon this interesting branch of surgery having yet appeared, the opinions of several professional friends have operated as an additional inducement in bringing forward some of the results of my own experience.

For the possession of most of the opportunities I have enjoyed, and for various facilities that have rendered them more valuable, I cannot forget that I stand principally indebted to Mr. HEAVISIDE, who, as surgeon to the St. George's Infirmary, has on various occasions given me much assistance; as well as by the communication of observations from the more immediate circle of his private practice.

It will be observed that I have been careful, particularly with regard to morbid structure, to distinguish what I have seen and examined with my own hand, from what has been stated upon the authority of others. This care seems necessary, having found that in circumstances relating even to the leading principles of pathology, error has occasionally crept in; and mere fancy, through the medium of generally received opinion, has at length assumed all the consequence of fact.

In the former edition, I selected those instances of disease of which I had then preserved the best notes. The opportunities I have since had of extending my experience have, I trust, enabled me to make in the present impression, some important additions; without giving me any reason to doubt the general correctness of the opinions previously brought forward. For some valuable and curious illustrations in the present edition, I am indebted to the friendly attention of Mr. SPILS-

BURY, of Walsall, in Staffordshire; whose zeal for the improvement of his profession is manifested by the readiness with which he kindly favoured me with the more recent fruits of his experience upon these subjects.* I have also taken the liberty to avail myself of such facts as appeared interesting, in looking over the few works that I have consulted; but in so doing have been careful not to omit acknowledging my obligations.

With regard to some circumstances contained in the following pages, it may perhaps be objected that the writer has wandered from his subject in adverting to complaints, the seat of which must evidently have been the superior parts of the alimentary canal. Upon this point the only apology he can offer is, that he was desirous of making these observations as really useful as possible, by rendering them practically so; and that he preferred the chance of censure for mentioning some particulars not precisely in order, to the omission of a single circumstance at all connected with the subject, which, being made known, may prove seriously important at the bed-side.

With relation to a very desirable object, the obtaining a regular habit of action in the bowels, which is rather a preventive than a curative measure, the author has ventured to propose and recommend a principle of treatment, that, as far as his reading extends, appears to have been little if at all, distinctly held in view by others. All that he can say in its favour is, that he has adop-

* See Cases 1. 2. 5. 6. 7. 12. 13. 14. 25. 63.

ted it in a great number of instances; and that, by little variations in the mode of its application, it has proved, with few exceptions, perfectly successful.

Upon some points it will be seen, that he has not hesitated to express opinions more or less at variance with those of surgeons of reputation and celebrity. If, however, this has been done with due regard to good manners, no apology can be necessary. It is by the collision of opinion that truth is elicited; and it will afford him infinite pleasure, should the present essay be considered in the least degree conducive to its developement.

PRACTICAL
OBSERVATIONS, &c.

CHAPTER I.

ON CONTRACTION, OR STRICTURE, IN THE RECTUM.

SECT. 1.

On the Causes of the Disease.

1. STRICTURE in the rectum may take place under various circumstances. Any accidental source of irritation in the bowels, any acrimonious secretion poured into the alimentary canal, or any extraneous substance detained in the lower part of the rectum, may, through the medium of inflammation, lay the foundation for this disease.

2. Where inflammation results from acrimonious matters in the bowels, its extent will usually be greater, and its consequences more serious, than when excited by the presence of an extraneous body.

I have, in one case, known a fish-bone lodged in the lower part of the rectum excite a very circumscribed spot of inflammation at the point most favourable for its escape near the verge of the anus; the ulcerated passage, upon the escape of the irritating cause, healing without any inconvenience to the future actions of the bowel.

I have, in many instances, while on service with the army, seen the most severe attacks of inflammation brought on, not only in the rectum, but along the superior part of the great intestine also, from the sudden accession of cholera morbus. Mere neglect of the bowels appears, in many instances, to have been the exciting cause of inflammation in the rectum, from the continual presence of acrimonious and bilious contents; where this action becomes chronic it either produces continued misery*, or worse consequences.†

3. When from any of the above causes inflammation in the bowel takes place, the natural texture being soft and vascular, the cavity of the affected part of the canal is apt to become diminished, and the thickness of its sides increased; and should the excitement principally affect the mucous membrane, coagulable lymph may be effused into the cavity of the bowel; this latter circumstance becoming in its turn a new cause of disturbance to the functions of the gut. If the irritation connected with the attack should prove violent, the above consequences may terminate in ulceration of the inner membrane of the bowel.

4. It has been believed by some surgeons, that stricture in the rectum may occur as the consequence of the venereal disease; but this opinion seems to rest on no better foundation than that of its having occasionally been met with in those who either had the misfortune to labour under both these complaints at the same time, or who

* Case 7. † Case 8.

had at least suffered from venereal disease at some former period.

5. The repulsion of eruptive complaints has been mentioned as a cause of this complaint, particularly by M. Desault, who relates two instances of it: I have seen several of a similar description.

6. It is probable that a disposition to contraction in the rectum may in some instances connect itself with hæmorrhoidal or fistulous complaints, and that the means adopted for the cure of the external disorder may appear to favour the subsequent advance of that which is internal, which had previously escaped without notice, or perhaps had not existed at all. My opinion upon this point is, that no operation for the cure either of hæmorrhoidal tumours, or fistulæ, ever did, or ever will, tend to the production of stricture or other disease of the gut, provided the operation is rightly performed, and that proper attention is afterward paid to the general health of the patient. The utter neglect of this latter circumstance I have very often seen bring on much inconvenience; and I know of a few instances in which it has cost the patient his life. We must not, however, discredit surgery unfairly, by imputing to it those events justly attributable to the neglect or ignorance of some few who practise it.

7. Stricture in the rectum sometimes occurs spontaneously, where it seems, notwithstanding, unfair to impute it to constitutional disease, as it comes forward alone, and yields readily to

treatment, provided that treatment is properly directed, and taken up in time.

8. The most serious, and indeed the only truly formidable shape in which this disease appears, is that in which it is commonly connected with some similar affection elsewhere, exciting symptoms, and exhibiting characters, that belong only to scirrhous disease: from which circumstance this particular variety of the complaint has been termed the malignant, scirrhous, or cancerous stricture of the rectum.

An interesting case of fatal stricture in the rectum, originating in cancerous disease of the womb, is related by Mr. WILMOT, in the second volume of that excellent work, the Transactions of the Irish College of Physicians.

9. M. DESAULT states that stricture in the rectum occurs less frequently in men than women, and this appears to be true, although I have not seen it in the proportion he has mentioned, of only one to ten.

10. Much inconvenience has sometimes arisen from a mere excess in the action of the sphincter muscle. M. DELPECH speaks of this circumstance as "un spasme fixe du muscle sphincter externe de l'anus, accompagne et peut-etre produit par une ou plusiers gercures placees dans les rides rayonnantes de cette ouverture."* One occasional consequence of spasm of this muscle will be mentioned presently (184.); and in a retention of urine which lately obliged me to puncture the bladder from the rectum, I found very considerable difficulty in passing my finger

* Precis. tom. i. p. 598.

through the sphincter, preparatory to making the puncture. It appeared that this spasm partly arose from the extreme pain and irritation kept up by the over-distended state of the bladder; particularly as in a preceding case in which I performed the same operation upon a gentleman then under my care for stricture, the introduction of the finger brought on great aggravation of the spasmodic pains in the bladder which repeatedly excited evident and distressing spasms in the sphincter.

Sect. 2.

On the Symptoms and Appearance of the Disease.

11. Inflammation in the rectum, excited by the presence of acrimonious matters within its cavity, is attended with feverish symptoms common to other local inflammations. In these affections I have generally observed tenesmus to be one of the most troublesome and constant sources of inquietude; particularly distressing, because the efforts to obtain relief are generally unavailing.*

12. A very usual, and sometimes strongly marked symptom, during inflammatory action in the lower part of the bowels, is a peculiar but decided sense of heat in the part affected.

Inflammation in the rectum may operate in some cases very formidably, by arresting the healthy functions of surrounding parts. In this way it may suspend the progress of labour†, and

* Cases 7. and 8.   † Case 5.

commonly produce retention of urine; or even a suspension of the secretion.*

13. Inflammation once produced, may vary in its progress and consequences. In strong and healthy constitutions, one of the most common ill effects is a degree of permanent thickening in the coats of the intestine, from serous fluid and coagulable lymph being poured out, either externally, internally, or into the cellular texture of the bowel. These events frequently end in the production of structure, sometimes in the formation of adhesions within the cavity of the gut, and occasionally in a permanent excess of irritability in the part, which it is next to impossible to relieve.

14. I have repeatedly known stricture in the rectum arise from coagulable lymph effused from inflammation connected with an abscess formed external to the gut. In one instance† the band of adhesive matter could be felt very distinctly in examining the bowel.

15. In the weak and irritable, though inflammation may end in effusion, the affection is more apt to run on to ulceration of the mucous membrane; and unless the probable state of the disease is accurately estimated, and the turn of constitution diligently attended to, the consequences will generally be serious, and the event fatal. Under these circumstances it commonly happens that the patient at first harrassed, is at last exhausted, by the combined influence of excessive secretion of purulent matter, long continued uneasiness, great pain, and incessant irritation.

* Case 6. † Case 11.

16. Where a fragment of a bone, or other sharp extraneous body, has found its way into the rectum, unless favourably situated for escaping by the sphincter, it usually excites inflammation and ulceration, by the aid of which it sometimes makes its way out; in other instances, however, this does not happen.

M. Le Dran mentions the laying open a fistulous sinus of many months' duration. In performing the operation, the surgeon, introducing his finger into the bottom of the wound, detected a small piece of bone with sharp edges, lodged very near the neck of the bladder. This was extracted, and the wound healed in two months.*

In one case, the jaw of a whiting was found at the bottom of an abscess near the anus, in a complaint previously supposed to be piles. It had subsisted more than a twelvemonth; but, on the removal of the cause, the abscess healed presently.†

In another case, an ivory bodkin, accidentally swallowed by a female, made its way from the intestines partially into the bladder; from whence, not without considerable difficulty, it was extracted, nine weeks afterwards, by making an opening into the bladder above the pubis.‡

Where an extraneous body is low down in the rectum, the patient is generally sensible of a sharp

---

* Observations de Chirurgie, Obs 86.
† Phil. Trans. No. 453.   ‡ Phil. Trans. No. 260.

prickling pain in the part, previous to the formation of matter, aggravated during the passage of a motion. Should he apply for assistance at this period, there will commonly be no difficulty in preventing the inflammation, or abscess, that otherwise must take place, by the timely removal of the irritating substance (48).

17. Inflammation, then, may be followed by permanent contraction or stricture, in the rectum. The inflammation removed, the coagulable lymph effused either between the coats, or into the cavity of the bowel, remains; and new-formed vessels shooting into its substance, enable it, slowly and imperfectly, to assume the characters of organized matter. The activity of circulation established in some of these newly-formed parts is such, that, instead of merely preserving their original form, they undergo a gradual increase or growth; and, provided the seat of the deposit be the cellular texture, the thickness of the sides of the bowel may increase, the aperture through the canal diminishing in the same proportion.

18. The attention of the patient is at length called to the state of the part affected. He suffers inconvenience or pain in passing a confined motion; he feels an irksome sense of weight, or bearing down; or, perhaps, is first struck by the appearance of a mucous discharge from the anus.

As the complaint increases, occasional difficulty or pain, when at the water closet, is succeeded by a progressive and generally an evident change in the form of every figured stool, which seldom fails, sooner or later, to point out the nature of the disease. The contents of the bowels have, in their appearance, been compared to thin flattened cords, or earth-worms.

19. By examining the bowel in the earliest or inflammatory stage, we ascertain the existence of extreme irritability, or severe pain, in the seat of the affection; the intestine feeling soft and pulpy, and the inner membrane thrown into folds.*

20. When the complaint has continued some time, and the sides of the gut are much thickened, in connection, perhaps, with effusion of coagulable lymph into the cavity, such thickening is more readily ascertained under examination. The lymph poured out into the canal may vary as to quantity and disposition: and, while recent, the adherent mass, whether divided into bands, or attached to one part only, may be peeled off, and separated by the end of the finger; or, if more perfectly organised, there are still other means by which its quantity may be lessened, or the inconveniences resulting from its presence removed.

Occasionally there are only a few small membranous septa passing across the canal, or a rough membranous surface, the extent of which may be determined by passing the finger on to the more perfectly smooth and elastic texture of the mucous membrane.†

In some cases stricture in the rectum is at-

---

* Case 4.   † Case 11.

tended with occasional sensations of sharp pain, at the end of the penis, similar to that which attends certain complaints in the bladder.*

21. When inflammation proceeds to ulcerate, the ulcerated surface will usually be very painful to the touch, and in some cases apt to bleed, unless, indeed, the cellular membrane has become sloughy. Should ulceration not have taken place, the thickening and consequent contraction in the coats of the canal will pass forward to the more advanced state of stricture, so as to prevent the introduction of the smallest bougie, and render the intestine at last impervious.

22. Where stricture in this part has been ascribed to the venereal disease, the complaint takes place in the manner above mentioned. The sides of the gut become thicker, and more firm than natural, lessening the diameter of the canal. It has been supposed that in this particular affection the mucous membrane of the bowel labours under an excitement similar to that which exists in the urethra in gonorrhœa; and to this circumstance the French writers have attributed the copious mucous discharges that occasionally attend the disease. I have, however, met with no fact in support of this opinion.

Should the disease have arisen from translation, or retrocession of cutaneous eruption, or should it be conceived to have originated in hæmorrhoidal or fistulous complaints, it will in either

---

* Cases 13. and 18.

case observe the course and exhibit the appearances already described.

23. The latter stages of strictured rectum, where it has no malignant tendency, are extremely distressing. The aperture of the stricture diminishing, the increased efforts required to expel the fæces become not only violent, but at length unavailing; while the urgent straining tends only to aggravate the irritation of the diseased parts, exposing the patient to a degree of misery and torment almost beyond description. Happily, however, even in these circumstances, the disease admits not only of being relieved but cured.

24. When the difficulties of the disease increase, it occasionally happens that abscess, takes place in the vicinity, which abscess, extending to the cavity of the intestine above the stricture, and opening externally also, allows the escape of at least some part of the contents of the overloaded intestines, a circumstance I had lately the opportunity of witnessing in a poor person, who, under much distress from this complaint, could not be prevailed on to allow the proper means to be used for her relief, and consequently fell a sacrifice to the disease. In a few instances an abscess of this kind has been known to form an opening from the bowel into the bladder, greatly aggravating the patient's general distress and misery.*

25. Of the malignant, scirrhous, or cancerous stricture, the early course frequently passes by

* Case 18.

without notice: it sometimes proceeds very slowly. In one case, the first symptoms was an occasional uneasiness, and frequent darting pain in passing a motion. In two other cases, one of which is annexed, the first symptom was an irritation at the neck of the bladder.* The more early symptoms are succeeded by those local inconveniences consequent to obstruction to the passage through the bowel.

26. The distinction between scirrhous stricture and contraction of any other kind, is always important, but not always easy; much assistance, however, may in general be derived from a careful attention to all the circumstances of the history.

It has been observed, that the firmness or induration in the feel of the stricture, and the apparently considerable extent of the affection, conveying the idea of a large mass fixed in the pelvis, is a criterion of its nature. This was once my opinion; but I have lately traced the same character in diseases from which, by proper care, the patients have perfectly recovered.

27. The symptoms I think most clear, are either a peculiar sharp pain darting through the seat of the disease, or a more constant sense of glowing warmth or heat in the part. These symptoms, as far as I have seen, attend only the malignant or scirrhous stricture. The means of relief also, as far as they relate to mechanical pressure, while they relieve other kinds of stricture, cannot be endured in this; they only tend to aggravate

* Case 20.

the symptoms, and hasten the progress of the disease.

28. The foregoing remarks relate to strictures so low down, as to be within the reach of operative surgery. Contraction of the bowels, however, may take place higher up, where no operation can avail. With regard to these cases, we have much to learn, as to the power of determining the seats and causes of disease, that we may be the better enabled to alleviate those complaints which may not admit of being entirely removed.

29. A case of stricture in the sigmoid flexure of the colon is recorded by Mr. HILL, which in its progress producing abscess in the rectum, and a fistulous opening into the membranous part of the urethra, terminated fatally after several years of distress and suffering; originating, as was supposed, in an injury received from a fall in hunting.* In another case by Dr. HOLMES, a stricture in the middle of the transverse arch of the colon was latterly attended with uneasiness in the abdomen, and an irritable loose state of the bowels.† For a very interesting case of this kind, the medical world are indebted to Dr. BURREL, in which stricture in the sigmoid flexure of the colon, terminating after a tedious and distressing illness in extensive ulceration through the coats of the bowel, ended fatally; which disease after death was found to have been produced by the poor man, who was a shoemaker, having accidentally swallowed five

---

* Edin. Med. Journal, vol. x.   † Ibid. vol. viii.

or six hogs' bristles, which in their passage had been stopped at that point, exciting disease not only there, but, by irritation, throughout the whole extent of the intestinal canal.*

In one remarkable case, stricture in the colon followed from a blow;† and within the last twelve months, I have had the care of an accident, in which a similar consequence would most probably have followed from a kick upon the abdomen, producing violent spasmodic and inflammatory pains in the situation of the transverse arch of the colon, and a copious as well as continued effusion of blood into the cavity of the intestine, with fever. By adopting the plan laid down for the treatment of inflammation (34.), the consequences of the accident were progressively removed, the patient felt relieved from the pain, the local tenderness, and lastly the difficulty in preserving an erect position; and in a few weeks considered himself in every respect perfectly recovered, giving reason to believe that the early attention paid to the injury was the means of preventing those more serious consequences which delay might have incurred.

30. Authors have attempted to distinguish the kind of stricture, by the state of the inner membrane. M. DELPECH states, that in the venereal stricture, the inner membrane becomes tubercular; most, but not all, instances in which I have found this membrane so changed, were clearly

---

* Edin. Med. Journal, vol. ix. † Case 22.

cases of scirrhus. M. DESAULT, more guarded, says that the inner membrane of the bowel occasionally acquires a surface more or less distinctly tubercular, whatever may be the nature of the stricture. The fact is, this tubercular state of the internal or mucous lining of the gut, arises generally, as far as I have examined the disease, either from the membrane becoming thickened, vascular, and pulpy from œdema; or from the contraction of the space within which it is confined, throwing it into numberless short, convoluted folds, and presenting a surface which the finger cannot well distinguish from a collection of soft tubercles.

31. The scirrhous stricture exhibits on dissection great and extensive thickening and consolidation, as well as confusion, of parts. The disease, not confined to the coats of the intestine, is continued more or less extensively into the cellular membrane beneath the peritoneum reflected over the sacrum, and bones of the pelvis. The firm, yet elastic, feel of this disease is peculiar, much resembling that of cartilage.

On opening the cavity of the bowel, the canal is found nearly or entirely closed, the section presenting so few traces of original structure as to render it difficult to say in what particular texture the disease originates. It appears to me to commence in the cellular membrane, connecting the coats of the intestine, an opinion not only rendered probable from the appearance of the parts, but from the evident facility with which the disease extends itself in the cellular tissue; it might also be argued from the tendency I have frequently remarked in scirrhous disease of the breast, to spread backwards, between the fibres of the pectoral muscle which can only happen by its affecting the cellular texture.

32. Where scirrhous stricture has ulcerated, the irritability of the disease being considerable, the ulcerative process in some instances makes rapid progress; the stricture, in fact, ceases to exist, for the lower part of the intestine is ulcerated through at various points: in this way an opening of communication is occasionally formed between the rectum and bladder.

A most interesting example, illustrative of this stage of the disease, is preserved in the Morbid Anatomical Collection of Dr. Hooper.

Sect. 3.

On the Treatment.

33. STRICTURE in the rectum may generally be prevented by an early and judicious attention to any inflammatory attack, to which this, no less than the other parts of the alimentary canal, is occasionally subjected.

34. Where inflammation is dependent upon acrimonious matters, plentiful dilution, by drinking copiously of light broths, or farinaceous decoctions, with repeated injections of warm water, will essentially tend to the relief and comfort of the patient, especially if assisted by the exhibition

of gentle aperients, neutral salines, and other diaphoretic medicines; together with the warm bath, if required. (92.)

35. The necessity or propriety of blood-letting will depend on the constitution of the patient, and the state of the pulse, as well as on the other symptoms. The pulse, although quick and hard, may not be sufficiently full to require, or to warrant, the abstraction of blood.

36. It is much to be lamented that in the treatment of internal diseases, their probable remote consequences are so little adverted to. The tendency of inflammation to produce effusion and contraction when it affects the urethra is now well known, but notwithstanding the other membranous and muscular canals are subject to the same law, it is not recognised; for when those events take place which almost invariably pave the way to the future production of stricture in the rectum, they are most commonly taken up on a wrong ground, or if present symptoms are relieved, no further precaution or enquiry is suggested, for none is thought of; although the readiness with which inflammation deposits coagulable lymph, and produces stricture in other canals, has been repeatedly explained, and is particularly unfolded in the valuable work of Sir EVERARD HOME on Stricture on the Urethra.

37. Regarding the consequences of inflammation in the urethra and in the rectum, as producing stricture, one material difference appears to be, the more frequent effusion of coagulable lymph

into the cavity of the canal in the latter, than in the former case.

Where adventitious adhesions have taken place in the rectum, their division ought to be effected, if within reach, but always with the least possible violence. If recent, the finger alone will be sufficient for separating them, without injury to the surface of the bowel. Where, however, force or violence is necessary, the division had better be made with a probe-pointed bistoury, or with scissars; the instrument being cautiously introduced upon the finger, without being suffered to pass beyond the reach of that best of all directors.

38. In the treatment of diseases, it is as important to be aware of those accidents that may favour us, as to be prepared for those that may be against us: it is therefore necessary to bear in mind, that an inflamed or strictureed' part of the bowel totally beyond the reach of the finger, may, through accidental circumstances, come at any moment completely within the power of examination; thus enabling the surgeon to satisfy himself most fully, as to figure, texture, and tendency.*

39. The occasional necessity for the aid of instruments, in dividing these adhesions, will be apparent, when it is recollected, that although coagulable lymph is easily separated or torn when it occurs as a recent deposit, its condition changes, it becomes organized, and the strength it

---

* Case 18.

may ultimately acquire is scarcely to be believed. In my practical observations in surgery, a case is related, in which the usual symptoms of hernia were produced by adhesions formed within the abdomen, strangling a part of the intestinal tube. It is difficult to conceive that any cord or band, the mere accidental result of effusion, should be capable of bringing about so serious a consequence. I was, however, lately requested to open the body of a young woman, in which examination I found the abdominal viscera in general much incommoded, and the omentum diseased, from inflammation, which had deposited various cords of coagulable lymph, connecting the bowels in various parts to each other, and to the pelvis. One of these cords, attached at one end to the anterior parietes of the abdomen, and the other to the small intestines, and thence indirectly to the spine, was scarcely thicker than a crow-quill, yet so strong, that raising it upon the fingers of both my hands, I found it strong enough to enable me to lift the body almost entirely from the table.

40. The great importance of being vigilant and prompt, with a view to the prevention of inflammation in the bowels, is more serious than is generally supposed. I have recently witnessed an instance in which adhesions from preceding inflammation caused infinite distress, and, after six years' incessant suffering, terminated fatally.*

* Case 21.

41. Considered practically, it is sometimes difficult to determine the precise extent, the seat, or even the actual presence of inflammation in the bowels. A degree of spasm will occasionally produce appearances and symptoms so closely resembling those of inflammatory action, that the distinction is almost impossible. The primary object, however, of these observations being to point out the means by which particular kinds of obstruction in the bowels may be effectually relieved, I think it right to mention my favourable opinion of a very powerful remedy, which I have known remove the most alarming degree of obstruction, where spasm presumably has been the cause. I have thrice had the opportunity of seeing its effects. They were cases in which the patients had suffered extreme pain in the region of the bowels, in which the prescriptions of physicians had availed nothing, and in which consequently Mr. HEAVISIDE's opinion and assistance had been requested; who, finding that the stomach had rejected every thing taken, and that stimulating clysters produced no favourable effect, in spite of bleeding, warm bath, and almost every other means, desired me to try the fume of tobacco, injected cautiously, by the proper apparatus, into the bowels. The usual effect of this application on the constitution is considerable lassitude and faintness, the pulse becoming much softer, and often irregular: it tends, of course, powerfully to relax any spasm in those parts to which it is most immediately applied; and it is curious that while it removes any excess of contraction in the

intestines, it manifestly excites a moderate diffused activity, producing a peculiar and remarkable disturbance, a general commotion and rumbling noise in the bowels, which, in each of the three cases to which I allude, was soon followed by copious evacuations of fæcal matter, and was evidently the efficient means of saving the life of the patient.

It may be objected that in the above cases the obstruction might not have been the consequence of spasm alone, but probably a degree of intussusception in some part of the bowels. To this it is only necessary to reply, that the obstruction being complete, the removal of it became, not only requisite, but essential to life, and that by the means employed the passage was restored, the pain removed, the feverish symptoms relieved, and the patient's life preserved.

42. Where spasm has produced obstinate constipation, the affusion of cold water has, under judicious management, been powerfully conducive to the removal of the constriction.*

43. Spasmodic contraction in various parts of the intestinal tube have occasionally given rise to very singular complaints; sometimes of a flatulent nature. Mr. COLLINS relates that a young woman, aged 17, had a tympanitic tumour presumably in the colon, which commenced as a small circular swelling in the right side, after several days of violent pain. It increased for near a twelvemonth, and had then reached the size of a quart basin

---

* Case 2.

in the centre, extending, laterally, almost the size of the arm, on each side, nearly round to the back. Steel medicines and purgatives were given without removing it. The affection was never painful, but inconvenient from distention. It never extended below the navel.*

In this case it is not easy to say how the bowel should or could have allowed the perpetual transit of the more solid contents of the canal without permitting the escape of the air also; provided it be admitted that the general cavity of the bowel was the seat of the collected flatus.

44. In some instances the retention of hard substances in the bowels, has excited spasm, and led eventually to the most serious consequences. An instance is on record, in which, after several years of complaint in the bowels, a single plum-stone was, after death, found to have quite burried itself, through the medium of ulceration in the villous coat, imbedding itself between the coats of the bowel, just where the colon joins the rectum. The part where this source of irritation lay was also found to be the seat of stricture, probably another effect of the irritation of the stone, which had produced a small abscess, discharging into the cavity of the pelvis, but not communicating with the canal of the intestine.†

45. The most extraordinary and curious instance, however, of this kind, that I have ever met with, was that of a female, who, at six years of age,

---

* Edin. Med. Journal, vol. i.   † Phil. Trans. vol. xxxix.

was first affected with a hard swelling and intense pain in the left side of the belly, which continned 12 hours, and subsided spontaneously. It returned, continued, and vanished, as at first, every three months; for several years; when the period of its return suddenly changed from three months to three weeks, and so continued till she was 85 years of age. At this time she married, and bore one child, the pain of child-brith being much less than that she had been accustomed to. Weak and exhausted by pain, watching, and the disappointment of finding that no medicine whatever relieved her, a woman gave her a strong dose of jalap, which operated very violently, removing the swelling (then the size of two fists) from the side, and driving the pain suddenly down from the side to the anus, where tenesmus, great forcing, and retention of urine, immediately came on.

Mr. YONGE, who relates the case, now called in, found a substance within the sphincter, which substance he extracted with the forceps, and permanently cured all her complaints. It was of an oblong figure, five inches in circumference, and although it weighed ten drachms, it swam on water. It was cut in two with a knife; externally it was black, as if coated with varnish; within this was a crust of matter like brick, as thick as half-a-crown; next to this appeared a substance resembling pasteboard or chewed paper: and within that a prune or withered plum, with the stone and kernel cut asunder by the knife.

" Thus all these surprising symptoms, that so

" long afflicted this poor woman, were occasion-
" ed by this plum, swallowed so many years be-
" fore; but how those different accretions were
" made to it in such a place as the intestines?—
" how it ceased to torment her at so many, and
" at such different intervals?—where it lurked
" between those fits, and how the pain and tu-
" mour observed such exact periods for so many
" years, at first every three months, and then
" every three weeks?—are questions I am not
" able to resolve."*

In the same volume of the work just referred to, several other cases are mentioned, where after repeated attacks of pain and spasm in the bowels, similar balls, each containing a plum-stone, have been passed per anum, the patient being either relieved or cured. Neither is it necessary that the substance should be hard, for a mass of strawberry-seeds retained in the bowels is stated, by Dr. SLOANE, to have in one instance produced as strange, and almost as obstinate, a distemper as he ever met with.

46. Even the more common fæcal matters, if permitted to remain in the bowels, will occasionally excite great derangement of health, without being even suspected as the cause. A woman is mentioned by PROFESSOR ODIER, who was subject to severe attacks of spasm, affecting, in a very peculiar manner, the circlating and respiratory organs, which were proved to have arisen from unheeded

---

* Phil. Trans. vol. xxiii.

confinement of bowels, and accumulation of fæces;* and I have myself repeatedly attended a lady in whom spasmodic attacks of pain, most agonising and frightful, seized upon the muscles of the loins and back, which, after continuing days and nights, (the bowels being stated to be perfectly regular,) have yielded to no medicines but cathartics, and to those only upon their producing from 20 to 30 copious, and fœtid stools. In this case there were no pains whatever in the bowels, and occasionally none in the affected muscles during a state of rest; but any attempt to turn in bed excited such torment as it was impossible to bear in silence.

A case of fatal obstruction in the bowels is recorded in the Philosophical Transactions,† in which the habitual difficulty in procuring stools was discovered, after death, to have originated in the lower end of the colon, folded back upon itself at a very acute angle, having formed a close adhesion for several inches along the line of contact.

In another case, a fatal ileus was produced in a boy, of which, in three days, he died, from an appendix, or hernions expansion of the bowel, three inches long, and as large as the bowel itself. Just below the insertion of this appendix, the intestine was so closely contracted by spasm as scarcely to admit the passage of a probe.‡

47. In considering the symptoms of inflammation in the rectum, it has been observed that the

---

* Edin. Med. Journal, vol. ii.
† No. 275.   ‡ Phil. Trans. vol. xliii.

probable consequences will much depend on the habit of the patient, and that notwithstanding the effects already noticed will commonly occur in strong constitutions, the weak and irritable will be more liable to suffer from another consequence, that of ulceration within the bowel. The probability of this event must be estimated by the small and deficient, though quick and even rapid pulse; by the state of the tongue varying towards the appearance observed in low typhoid fever; and by other characters of weakness or irritation. Examination of the bowel conveys some information; there is little disposition to contraction, combined with great local irritability.

48. Of inflammation from local irritation, I have known two instances in which a fish-bone, escaping into the throat, has, through inflammation, produced stricture in the œsophagus, creating much inconvenience to the patient: although in one of these I know it did not shorten life, as the patient lived many years afterwards, and then died from some other cause. In one case, I have found a small bone passed through the intestines give rise to very unpleasant consequences in the rectum, producing an abscess, which, although it eventually allowed the escape of the irritating substance, left an unhealthy state of parts, that required time and attention to remove.

49. A gentleman applied to me with uneasiness and pain in the rectum, which he could not explain: suspecting some local irritation, I examined, and found the sharp edge of rather a large

fragment of bone pressing against the sides of the bowel. He was requested to return home, and remain quiet in bed, where, with the assistance of some spongetent, I succeeded in relaxing the sphincter sufficiently to introduce two of my fingers. By this means the extraneous body, which had already excited much irritation, was safely removed, and further mischief prevented.

50. The treatment of stricture in the rectum cannot be taken up too early. The contracted part, provided the mischief has not proceeded far, may admit the finger to pass freely through, without giving any distinct impression of coagulable lymph within the cavity, or of ulceration of the mucous membrane.

In this state, the common wax bougie, or perhaps, in preference, one of elastic gum of moderate size, may be introduced through the stricture, and allowed to remain or not, according to circumstances. If the parts are irritable, they must be quieted and humoured; if otherwise, they may be treated with less reserve.

51. The frequency of passing an instrument must be regulated by the state of the parts; the operation may usually be repeated at least every few days. It will require some knowledge of these complaints to determine whether the complaint is in a state that is favourable for the use of the bougie. Where the least tendency to inflammatory action exists, I have known the symptoms much aggravated by a single application of this kind; whereas, had due attention and discernment been

shown regarding the previous state of the parts, they might, by the direction of proper medicines, have been easily brought into a state more favourable for operating, saving the surgeon much loss of time, and the patient much unnecessary pain. The want of attention to this principle in treatment is, I am convinced, frequently productive of great misery. A patient I lately had, complained, when he gave me the history of his disorder, that one of the surgeons who had previously attended him had put him to extreme torture in using the bougie, a circumstance which must have favoured the formation of a large abscess found after death, which from the symptoms, appeared to have existed long before he first applied to me.[*]

52. Where contraction from inflammation becomes established, or rather makes a slow and steady progress, the necessary treatment may prove tedious, but the event, under proper management, is almost sure of being favourable. The introduction of the bougie may be required every day, or it may be necessary to increase its diameter more quickly than common, in order to gain upon the disease: or it may be expedient, with a view to excite absorption of the newly deposited matter, that the operation be so conducted as to produce, and keep up, a certain degree of pain, or at least uneasiness, during the continuance of the pressure.

53. All these circumstances must be regulated by the discretion and judgment of the practitioner:

---

[*] Case 18.

one point being so balanced against another as may afford the best prospect of ultimate, success, by promoting absorption, and favouring relaxation. That absorption may reasonably be expected to take place, by adoption of the plan proposed, is sufficiently proved by the frequency with which we see it excited by the agency of pressure, under other circumstances. At all events it is most true, that I have, in many cases, found the thickening diminish, the induration decrease, the aperture of the stricture enlarge, and the patient made most happy, without any other assistance than which the judicious application of the bougie has afforded.

54. Stricture in the rectum, when supposed to be connected with venereal complaints, has exhibited no distinct or peculiar symptoms; and those who have advocated such connection have admitted that the only mode of determining the point is by placing the patient under the influence of mercury, which, say they, if the complaint is venereal, will effect a cure.

55. Should the disease advance, the aperture through the stricture becomes progressively lessened, till at length the mechanical obstruction, at first occasional, is now constant, with aggravated suffering, and increased distress. The frequency of desire to pass a motion, the difficulty in effecting its passage, and the degree of pain brought on by the attempt, become almost insupportable. The treatment, however, is to be still conducted upon the principles already laid down.

56. In dilating strictures of this kind, M. DE-SAULT was in the habit of introducing a slip of lint, passed upon a probe through the strictured part, and allowed to remain there some time. In the course of the treatment, the quantity of lint thus introduced was increased, so as to answer the same purpose as a series of bougies; and the plan consequently proved as successful as that of introducing the bougie. I have repeatedly tried both modes, and certainly prefer the bougie; this instrument presents a more perfectly smooth surface, gives much less pain in the introduction, and, as far as my experience goes, has answered the purpose better than the other method.

57. The disease now under consideration, it might naturally be concluded, could not, in any instance, pass through all its stages without exciting attention; but the degree of indifference manifested in some instances regarding health is scarcely credible. I was, some months back, shown a disease just removed by a medical friend from the body of a lady, fifty years of age, who died in the country. She had never applied for any opinion upon her case till a week previous to her disease, when, complaining of confined bowels, she requested her apothecary to send her some medicine. Large doses of the sub-muriate of mercury, and other powerful purgatives, were given without effect; injections were adminstered, but could not be made to pass. Violent pains soon came on in the bowels, and continued till she died. On opening the body, part of the small. and the whole

of the large intestines were found loaded with fluid and fæcal matter, and very much inflamed. The cause of the obstruction was discovered low down in the pelvis, near the termination of the rectum, where gut had become so nearly impervious from stricture, as to prevent the introduction of any but the smallest sized probe.

58. Abscess in the vicinity of the stricture usually allows the escape of a part of the contents of the bowels. When, however, the stricture is relieved, and the natural passage partly restored, the fistulous channel generally assumes a healthy disposition, and soon closes up, similar to what happens in fistula in perinæo, from stricture of the urethra. Where, on the other hand, the removal of the obstruction in the bowel is not followed by the healing up of the fistulous passage, the partial or complete division of it will be all that is required for perfecting the cure.

59. In scirrhous stricture, it has been already observed, that pressure does harm; and, as the application of the bougie is therefore out of question, we are obliged to rest upon those palliative measures which consist in the direction of proper medicines, these, under judicious regulation, will often afford relief and comfort, although they may leave us in uncertainty as to the event of the disease.

60. M. DELPECH says, that where the advanced state of the disease precludes the passage of the fæces, it has been proposed to divide the strictured gut, to secure the escape of the contents of the

bowels, the confinement of which must, of course, produce extreme distress and danger. He adds, that the carrying up a cutting instrument into the midst of a cancerous disease must be expected to produce ulceration, and, in this way, hasten the destruction of the patient; but that, in cases of this kind, every thing that can be proposed is subject to objection. His words are: "On "a propose de faire alors la section de l'un de "ces points intermediares, afin d'assurer le pass- "age des matieres. Ce parti a de grande iucon- "veniens sans doute. Porter l'instrument tran- "chant au milieu ou tout pres d'une affection "cancereuse, c'est hater l'ulceration, qui doit "consommer la ruine du malade; mais dans des "cas de cette nature, on ne peut rien entreprendre "que de tres defectueux."* Upon this point I must take the liberty to observe, it appears to me that operative surgery should rarely, if ever be recommended, unless where the chances are decidedly in favour of its success; and if this opinion is right, it must unquestionably be wrong to advise an operation in a disease of inevitably fatal event. It can only tend to discredit that branch of surgical practice, which, from the positive good that, properly directed, it is capable of conferring, lays the fairest claim to the regard and confidence of mankind.

61. From its known power of allaying irritation, opium, in the latter stages of scirrhous stricture, becomes our chief dependance and the principal

* Précis Elementaire, tom. iii. p. 559.

means of relief, assisted occasionally by other medicines of the same class. The distressing sensations experienced in the parts may sometimes be alleviated by the introduction of suppositories of the extract of opium, of conium, or of hyoscyamus, singly or combined, according to circumstances. One advantage attributed to suppositories is, that the application made in a solid form dissolves slowly, and thus operates more in the manner of a permanent remedy. In one patient, however, whom I some time since attended, a suppository of opium, directed to be introduced with this view gave much additional uneasiness, and that repeatedly; but the same quantity of opium, dissolved in a warm injection, had an excellent effect, and was always productive of much relief, and very great, though temporary, comfort.

62. The treatment of contraction from spasm of the sphincter, must be regulated by circumstances. In the cases mentioned by M. DELPECH, the attempts made to dilate the parts increased the distress, and did harm. But the description given certainly implies the existence of some venereal taint in the habit, to correct which, as it appears to me, should have been the first step. That gentleman, however, advises that the stricture be removed, by carrying a free incision through the fibres of the muscle, taking care so to heal the wound as to prevent the re-union of the divided parts. This operation, I confess, I have never seen performed, and, as a matter of opinion, should think very rarely necessary.

Case 1.

Obstruction of the Bowels with suspected Stricture.

A gentleman, between forty and fifty, much addicted to the pleasure of the palate, has had several serious attacks within the last few years, of loaded and obstructed bowels. These complaints have been ushered in by restlessness, nausea, epigastric fulness, tension and soreness in the lower part of the abdomen, and acute pain on pressure. In the attacks, the tongue was pale white, with a brown granulated fur on the basis; the pulse accelerated, with total loss of appetite, and a slight bilious tinge in the conjunctive membrane of the eyes. He complained that his stools were in general ejected with violence, preceded by wind. The first application of purgatives produced a pitchy feculence, scalding, and irritating, and, by degrees, the bowels, naturally very torpid, yielded a slimy evacuation of highly concentrated green bilious matter. Occasionally these latter are interrupted by the pitchy secretion, with increase of the symptoms. The nights are sleepless with pain in the back, and irritable sensations in the limbs. The evacuations indicate no deficiency of bilious secretion, but an excess of a highly odorous pitchy feculence, alternating with slimy yellow flocculent matter. Steady and sedulous perseverance in laxatives, opiates, alkaline infusions, with clysters, gradually bring the patient from a state of danger to one of comparative ease and recovery. By means of a small rush-light candle, no bougie being at hand, I examined the state of the rectum. About six inches from the sphincter I met with an obstruction. Gentle pressure seemed to admit the end suddenly through a diminished aperture, with pain and faintness, the patient saying that he felt an increase of the pain in his back.

Since this period he has been disinclined to have the bougie passed, so that although I have little doubt of stricture being present, I cannot, without more clear evidence, decide positively upon its existence.

I have seen a figured stool: it is small, about the size of a child's motion.

Case 2.

Obstinate Constipation of Bowels.

B. T., aged thirty, had symptoms of an inflammatory affection of the bowels from June 3. to July 21, 1819. He had much fever, and tenderness on pressure, and irritation at stomach, with hepatic excitement; which yielded to bleeding general and local, purgatives, blisters, and anodynes.

He passed through July and August with restless nights, without appetite, and almost without strength; when he was advised change of air. By this assistance he became well, and returned to his occupation of a bit-maker, in better health than he had enjoyed some time.

May 7, 1820. I was called to him, he was labouring under great tension of the abdomen, vomiting, anxious restlessness, and excessive pain referred to the lower bowels and back; and although he had taken castor-oil repeatedly for several days, he could scarce procure any evaenation. I bled him to the amount of twenty ounces, with relief to the rapidity of the pulse, the vomiting and pain. An injection was next administered of turpentine and castor-oil, in a full quart of gruel. Draughts, with castor-oil and tincture of rhubarb, were also given every two hours.

8. No evacuation; tensive bowels. The injection had partly stayed, and was now repeated. Twenty leeches were applied to the belly. A scruple of calomel, with a purging mixture, given every hour, and a blister laid upon the abdomen. Only the injection returned, no fæcal matter.

9. Nine more leeches were applied to the circumscribed tumid part of the colon, near the sigmoid flexure, but still no evacuation. I now wished to try the tobacco glyster; but as no apparatus for the fume was at hand, a scruple was given infused for ten minutes. It produced deathlike prostration of strength, but no stool; it was repeated with as little effect; and also a third time, but still no evacuation.

11. Seven in the morning, still without evacuation. I had my patient taken out of bed, supported, and a couple of gallons of cold water

dashed violently over the abdominal region. He was rubbed dry, a tobacco glyster administered, and then put to bed. I left directions, that if no evacuation occurred before noon, another glyster from an infusion of a drachm and a half of tobacco, should be given. This was done. Half-past 10 at night I visited him, and had the pleasure to find him in comfort and safety. His bowels had given way about six in the evening, and he had had three or four copious evacuations. Sound sleep followed; and by the twentieth of the month he was perfectly couvalescent.

The pain and restlessness were much relieved by the depletion, but the anxiety and want of sleep were by no means allayed. As far as the patient's own feelings might be trusted, he considered the cold water as having produced the change in the state of his bowels, for they had made more disturbance on that day; probably the fortunate result may be attributed to the conjoint effect of the treatment.

Case 3.

Inflammation of the Rectum.

A stout young woman, aged twenty-two, complained of heat and pain about the rectum and anus, April 3. She said, that an anxiety to keep her place had induced her to conceal her ill health as long as she could. Her bowels were confined, her pulse quickened, and her skin hot; she complained of constant burning heat internally, extending from the fundament several inches along the bowel; connected with which, there was heat and tumour in the perineum. She was ordered some opening medicine, but neglected taking it; and on the following day was ordered fomentations, being much worse.

April 5. I was requested to see her. She complained principally of the great heat and constant sense of burning, extending several inches along the intestine, connected with so much external swelling and inflammation below the right labium, as to preclude more particular examination. With a very white tongue, and a hot and dry skin, she had much thirst, and a pulse at 120.

The fomentations were continued, and four large leeches applied to the perineum; but the pain not being at all relieved, eight ounces of blood were extracted by cupping as near the part as possible. By these means, the internal sense of heat and pain in the rectum immediately gave way, and in a few hours was quite gone; the external heat, pain, and swelling, remained, for which, fomentations, rest, and low diet, were directed.

On the following day (the 6th) she took castor-oil, which brought away several highly offensive stools, to her great relief; the fomentations were continued.

April 7. In the course of this afternoon, the abscess in the perineum broke, the discharge from which was intolerably fœtid. She found immediate relief, and by the next day was quite easy, but very weak. As the fever now left her, she took bark, and within a fortnight the abscess was healed, and she was perfectly recovered.

Case 4.

Inflammation of the Rectum.

Jan. 12. 1819. I was consulted by a gentleman of delicate habit, for a complaint in the rectum. He said that about five weeks before, he had contracted a very slight gonorrhœa; that being confined in his bowels, he a few days afterward felt pain in passing his motions, which complaint had now become very distressing. The pains were occasional and acute, either confined to the bowel, near the anus, or shooting thence upwards to the loins. There was a constant, though variable sense of heat in the part; the passing a motion was extremely painful, especially just afterward, exciting tenesmus, and irritation at the neck of the bladder. The examintion of the rectum gave excessive pain, exciting the most violent nervous agitation; the feel of the bowel was that of an irritable and thickened, but, at the same time, a spongy and relaxed part; the temperature was evidently raised above the natural standard; there was nothing amiss with the prostrate, but gentle pressure towards the sacrum instantly brought on the peculiar pain in the loins of which he had complained, as if the state of the bowel had connected itself with some affection of the sacral nerves: the tongue was white; the pulse at 90, small, but hard. There was a trifling appearance of discharge from the urethra, but an elastic gum bougie passed with freedom, and without pain. He was directed to keep quiet, live low, and take gentle aperients to procure three or four motions daily. From this plan he experienced some relief.

Jan. 15. He had been very poorly, with constant irritation and distress about the loins and rectum. He was ordered some castor-oil, which, with other medicines, procured several copious stools, and so much relief, that by the next morning he was easy and comfortable.

Jan. 17. He was not quite so well, the tongue still covered with a thick white crust; the pulse still at 90; the skin hot, and thirst considerable. The apparent state of the bowel, on examination, much the same: pressure externally, above the pubes, gave no uneasiness. I now directed the saline draught, with tincture of opium, to be taken every four hours.

Jan. 19. By the assistance of aperients, copious fæcal evacuations were obtained, and the symptoms much relieved. The tongue became cleaner, and the pulse soft, and reduced to 80. The medicines were continued.

Jan. 23. His complaint had quite left him, but he was very weak. It was, however, considered prudent to allow him to recover his strength slowly; the aperient medicines, therefore, were continued, but he was directed to take light nourishment more freely than before. Under this plan he soon entirely recovered.

Feb. 12. On examination, the bowel was ascertained to be in every respect restored to its natural state.

Case 5.

Inflammation of the Rectum; retarding Labour.

I was sent for to attend a Mrs. S. aged forty, with her first child. I found her in excessive irritation, referring all her pain to a constant sense of violent bearing down, and uneasiness in the rectum. She had been in labour three days, and about ten days before, coming home at night, she fell in the dark, and hurt herself. For a week after the accident she had scarcely any motion, but the continual and dreadful pain in and above the fundament, was the cause of all her sufferings. On examining the os uteri, the labour was found to be natural, and coming forward. On passing the finger into the rectum, though the bulk of the head pressed there, yet the finger could get beyond, and the gut did not seem to be unusually compressed, certainly not sufficiently to account for the great uneasiness in the bowel, which superseded the regular pains of uterine action. With head-ach, wandering pains, accelerated vibrating pulse, and a brown parched tongue, she was directed some opening medicine without effect, an aperient injection also was administered without operating to her relief. The patient seemed to be in great danger. I immediately took away fourteen ounces of blood; in half an hour the uneasiness in the rectum grew more tolerable, the pain in the head was relieved, the wandering pains ceased, and the uterus exerted its full power, the pains becoming regular, with intervals of ease.

In about three hours, during which I staid with her, she felt great comparative relief and comfort; and sat up cheerfully when I left her.

In the morning I found the pains had been regular, the labour advancing, but still complaints of the rectum; though not near so intolerable as before. At about two o'clock she was delivered of a dead child. By brisk cathartics, and occasionally an anodyne, she recovered speedily.

The whole of this case may be considered as having been untoward and protracted, by the medical gentleman, whom I did not know was attending until afterwards, not being aware of the inflammatory state, rendering the case complicated.

Case 6.

Inflammation of the Rectum; with Retention of Urine.

I was called to visit a young man with constipated bowels, and retention of urine. He could neither pass his water, or had he the power of going to stool, although the inclination to both was urgent, and very painful.

His pulse was full and hard, and as he had not been in this state a great number of hours, I blooded him until syncope came on; very shortly after which he felt greatly relieved from the painful state of rectum, and also in the bladder. Both the bladder and intestines were soon after emptied of their contents upon the operation of a brisk purgative, which completed his comfort and recovery.

Case 7.

Chronic Inflammation of Rectum; mistaken for Piles.

A lady, lately confined, had just gotten down stairs, but still annoyed with a severe pain in the rectum. She had suffered frequently on going to stool, during the greater part of her pregnancy, but now has expressed such dread of going to the water-closet, that her life was quite burthensome. She had complained to her medical attendant, who assured her it was piles, which a little castor-oil would remove. Her sufferings, however continned, and she was brought in fainting from the water-closet, when my attendance was requested. I learned that her stools were scanty, but that she always experienced the greatest excess of pain in passing her motions. Her general health pretty good, she was not much inconvenienced when free from severe pain. On examining the rectum, I found it filled with hard lumps: I extricated as much as I could with my finger. Clysters were then employed, with active laxatives. The colon and rectum were successively emptied; in a very few days she was perfectly free from any complaint, and has remained so ever since, now many months.

Case 8.

Diseased Rectum, from Inflammation.

Dec. 30. 1820. I was desired by Mr. HARDY, surgeon of Wolworth, to visit a patient, a middle-aged man, who, for years, had been subject to bilious attacks in the bowels, at first occasional, but latterly so frequent that he at length totally neglected them; and during the months of September and October last, was distressed by a complaint for which he did not even seek relief. He had experienced a contant desire, night and day, to be on the night-chair, and had no sooner left it than the desire returned, with scarcely the power to pass any thing, except a little thin slime, or sometimes a bit of hardened fæces, with a continual and distressing sense of heat and uneasiness in the rectum, feverish restlessness, and thirst.

In November he requested Mr. HARDY to see him, who directed various opiates and anodynes, to soothe and compose his feelings; and his medicines much relieved him. The motions, of late, when consistent, had been observed to be apparently small in diameter, leading to suspicion of stricture. A pill of colocynth and calomel was what seemed to answer best in regulating the bowels; and, to allay the irritation in the rectum, a pill of extract of poppies, and extract of hyoscyamus, of each three grains, to be taken every six hours

The above is the outline of the case, with which Mr. HARDY kindly furnished me. On enquiry, he said he had never had the least uneasiness, or affection of bladder, but a great and distressing sense of weight very low down in the bowel.

On examination, there was no appearance of external disease. Within the sphincter I found the bowel not at all contracted, but on the contrary, its capacity was pretty evidently increased, yet completely altered from its natural state. In parts it was firmly adherent to the sacrum, posteriorly, and laterally, having large firm folds, or ridges, passing in various directions; not feeling at all as if lymph had been effused into the cavity, but between the coats of the bowel. Upon reflection, the peculiar position of the case enabled me to explain what was new to me, by perceiving that the attack of inflammation must have taken place at a time when the rectum was very much loaded; a circumstance which, in a neglected and costive habit, might easily occur; and that the spaces between the masses of hardened fæces had determined the particular cast and figure of the internal surface of the bowel, upon the consolidation of the fluid poured out between its coats.

In consultation, it was determined to continue his medicine, with the addition of an occasioual injection of warm gruel, containing thirty drops of laudanum.

Jan. 8. 1821. The medicines had been useful, the injection had afforded him comfort, and, upon the whole, he thought himself somewhat better. As the particular object of this visit was to make a more perfect examination of the bowel, an aperient having operated, the rectum was first injected with warm water; and a large-sized silver ball, then introduced, was passed progressively and easily forward, until it reached a natural turn of the intestine. On its removal, the instrument was found to have traversed an extent equal to ten inches, to which extent the bowel was perfectly sound, except in the part already mentioned.

It was considered advisable to continue the medical treatment, upon the principle already acted on; there being no ground for recommending other means.

Case 9.

Stricture of the Rectum, from Inflammation.

L. R., aged thirty, had inflammation and abscess at the side of the rectum, in the year 1809, followed by two years' ill health and two operations for fistula. At the close of this period, she felt increased pain in going to stool, and had a considerable mucous discharge from the rectum and vagina. Medical assistance improved her general health, but she requested admission into St. George's Infirmary, in December, 1811. On examination, I found a contraction, like a thin membranous circle, about two inches within the anus, which appeared to me an affection of the mucous membrane alone. It seemed a very fair case for the application of the argentum nitratum, which, I have no doubt, would have cured her, but she objected to it. Repeated trials having proved that the irritability of the parts was too great to admit of her deriving benefit from the unarmed bougie, she left the house. A more particular detail of this case is given in the Surgical Observations.

Case 10.

Stricture in the Rectum.

In Nov. 1811, I operated for fistula in ano upon a lady aged twenty-eight; the wound healed readily. In February following, I was again consulted for a difficulty occasionally observed in passing her motions. This complaint was inconvenient or distressing, according to the state of her bowels.

On examination, the intestine was found contracted, but so high up, that the part where the stricture was greatest, was beyond the reach of the finger. The gut was not apparently much thickened, nor at all confined laterally: these points were favourable, although the strictured part was extremely irritable. The examination gave much pain, exciting great nervous agitation. She was advised to allow a bougie to be passed; and two days afterwards this was done: a wax bougie, of moderate size, curved to the course of the bowel, was introduced. It was with some difficulty, and very severe pain, that the instrument passed the seat of the contraction; allowed to remain, the pain became easier, but was increased by the withdrawing the bougie, the stricture grasping it very closely. A composing draught was directed to be taken immediately.

The same instrument passed twice a week, for six weeks, so essentially relieved the complaint, (the bougie passing with so much less resistance, and the motions with so much more ease and freedom,) that it was proposed to introduce one that was a size larger; but as the patient now found herself perfectly free from all the symptoms to which the stricture had given rise, she preferred waiting to see whether she might not remain well, without further assistance.

Since the above period, there has been no return of the complaint.

Case 11.

Stricture, from Inflammation of the Rectum.

J. W., a servant, aged thirty-two, in October, 1818, slipped in descending some steps, and received a violent contusion upon the perineum. Severe pain and inflammation followed; she, however, continued to do her work.

In the course of a month, no longer able to move, she kept her bed, mentioned the accident, and was advised to poultice and foment; soon after which, the extreme heat, pain, and swelling were relieved by something breaking, as she thought, into the bowel; and the opinion was confirmed by the flow of a copious purulent discharge from the anus: the same kind of matter was, after this, passed constantly with her motions.

Dec. 1. She came into the St. George's Infirmary: fomentations and poultices were continued till January 2., when the abscess opened externally, near the anus. The same treatment was still continued.

In examining the parts, January 23., I found, on the left of the sphincter, some extent of integument detached, perforated in several places, and discharging pus. The verge of the anus was concealed by what seemed hœmorrhoidal tumours, but by their puffy flaccid feel, were ascertained to be only an œdema of the cellular membrane. Passing the finger per anum, I found that what she said as to difficulty in voiding her motions was correct. For an inch and a half the bowel was unaltered; above this an obstruction existed. It was a defined circular ring, formed within the intestine, not at all resembling the feel of the smooth, soft, inner membrane. It firmly adhered to the cavity, and had a contracted central opening, through which, with some little pressure, and complaint of pain, I passed my finger, perceiving at the instant a partial laceration of its substance. The stricture was thus ascertained to be not quite two inches in extent, beyond which the bowel was healthy.

The feel of this adventitious substance was very different from that of any originally formed stricture: it was peculiarly rough, spongy, somewhat fragile, and capable of being partially detached. A probe, introduced by one of the external openings, discovered a sinus, leading near five inches along the outside of the intestine; the structure, however, prevented my being able distinctly to feel the point of the probe.

Jan. 26. She said she had been able to pass her stools better since the examination. As a first step in ascertaining the exact tone of the parts, a bougie of tallow was passed through the stricture, and allowed to waste, by the warmth and action of the surrounding parts, a plan that Mr. HEAVISIDE is partial to as possessing several advantages. It certainly determines the present measure of irritability very accurately, without the risk of increasing it, as the wasting of the bougie is in effect equivalent to its removal, without the disturbance incident to its being withdrawn.

Jan. 30. The same application was repeated.

Feb. 2. A bougie of wax, rather less than the former, covered with oiled lint, was passed through the stricture. This produced increased pain, appearing to depend more on the roughness of surface, than the size of the instrument. It was expected this circumstance might prove an advantage, but it seemed to operate rather unfavourably, creating too much pain and disturbance.

Feb. 6. and 9. The same bougie alone was passed; the operation was much less distressing, and apparently more beneficial, by allowing the parts to remain quiet.

Feb. 15. A bougie of larger size, of elastic gum, was introduced; it passed with great facility, although, from dilating the stricture, it excited an aching pain during the half hour it was allowed to remain. On the 17th and 19th the operation was repeated. On the 23d, I laid open the sinus leading up by the side of the intestine, dressing it with lint, as in the operation for fistula.

March 9. With copious suppuration, and more pain, a slight attack of erysipelatous inflammation came upon the perineum, with tremors, and feverish heat. The rectum, on examination, was found heated, but the circular band of coagulable lymph, though somewhat more contracted, was not perceptibly more firm than before; the bowel beyond the stricture was still in its natural and healthy state.

For these complaints she was directed to foment, and take the bark with sulphuric acid. These means were continued till April 8., when, being quite recovered from the attack of inflammation, and much improved in strength, she was recommended to try the cold bath, the discharge being still rather considerable. The cold bath proved rather too powerful, and it was therefore re-peated locally. The internal use of tonics, and the regular introduction of the bougie, were now continued on to the 20th of April, when a very large-sized bougie passed with perfect ease, and the discharge had nearly ceased. She now felt herself sufficiently recovered to propose leaving the Infirmary and returning to service, since which she has remained well.

Case 12.

Stricture of the Rectum; mistaken for Dyspepsia.

An elderly man, upwards of fifty, complained of pain, load and uneasiness at stomach, he was restless, his eyes suffused with a bilious tinge, yet the evacuations were sufficiently coloured with bile. His health was rather improved by taking a laxative pill of rhubarb, ipecacuanha, and divided doses of calumba and soda. He had before placed himself under medical treatment for the same complaint of stomach, supposed to be his only disorder; at that time alteratives and bitter infusions seemed to relieve him; but the returning attacks became more severe and obstinate.

In process of time his nights became restless, but having had a suspicious correction he became alarmed and could not be persuaded the weariness in his limbs, shooting and lacinating pains in the groins, numbness in the scrotum, and pain in the urethra and back, were attributable to any thing but infection. He would hardly listen to the suggestion of any other cause, until I explained that the secondary symptoms of lues had a primary affection certain and unerring in character. The bladder sounded, was found in a healthy state; the urethra without stricture. On introducing my finger in the rectum I found the entrance narrow, snd a little way in the walls somewhat thickened, but no stricture within reach; the prostate was much enlarged. I oiled and passed a small rectum bougie; at the distance of about six inches resistance was found, but on a little pressure the point advanced, when immediately both groins were seized with lancinating pains. It required some days to allay the irritation from the cautious use of the bougie. At present his plan of treatment is confined to palliative means, the application of the bougie being evidently improper.

Case 9.

Stricture of the Rectum.

A man aged 35, came to consult me almost in despair, for venereal symptoms. His distress was occasioned by constant pain, referred to the end of the penis, with uneasiness about the scrotum. He had been under the care of three medical men all of whom had mercurialized him either by pill or potion for this said lues; at last one sagaciously observed, if it was it, he had taken medicine enough to cure a dozen, and that he really did not know what to do with him.

In this state he came to me, but neither by his own account or by examination could I deteet his having had a single venereal symptom. His fears had been excited, and appeared to have been taken advantage of, for each of his attendants, for a period longer or shorter, had put him under the venereal treatment. The bladder was sounded, without discovering stone, or stricture; but the pain and heaviness in the loins led me to examine the rectum, when about five inches above the sphincter a stricture was discovered.

By the use of bougies, the pains and other symptoms in a great measure ceased, but an attack of rheumatic fever has for the present set aside the continuance of the necessary local treatment.

Case 16.

Stricture in the Rectum.

An elderly woman had long complained although with no distinct evidence of bad health. She either assigned her occasional paroxysms of pain in the back to rheumatism, or gravel; when it was thought to be rheumatism, it was treated with a strengthening plaster; when gravel, by gin and water at bed-time. Her paroxysms became more severe, the occasional expulsion of wind from the stomach was assisted more frequently, and by necessity, with ginger and mint tea. Loss of flesh and restlessness required larger doses of a composing electuary; so that her life was occupied in ringing the changes, on wind, rheumatism, and gravel.

Not exactly satisfied with her urgency that she knew her complaints and remedies, but, with significant hints that she was a martyr to her husband, I made an examination of the rectum, and immediately within the sphincter found the gut contracted, exhibiting to the feel an indurated hard tenches mouth, which the point of the little finger would not enter. The poor woman would not submit to any treatment, but still insisted on her imaginary diseases; and for the last few months has been in a declining and sinking state.

CASE 15.

Stricture in the Rectum.

Jan. 5. 1821. A middle aged gentleman visited me, having come from Cambridge for my opinion, upon a complaint that he said by some had been considered mental, by others corporeal, and by some few a mixture of both together. He had of late been extremely annoyed by flatulent complaints in the bowels, and an uneasy sense of tightness in the abdomen: now and then to spasmodic pains in one or other part of the intestines. Purgative medicines he had frequently used, and at first they were beneficial, but latterly they not only failed to relieve by relaxing, but invariably created additional distress, by aggravating the uneasiness, pain, and flatulence. He said no one had enquired into the existence of any local complaint. He had consulted one physician who belonged to the university, who considering the disorder dependant on weakness, had prescribed for him, without benefit. He had also seen a physician of high reputation in London, who told him his complaint was indigestion, and that his prescription would cure him presently, but it did nothing. Usually his bowels were relaxed, but he never seemed relieved, nor ever felt as if his intestines were fairly emptied; even when he had frequent motions. Occasionally, when his bowels were somewhat confined, he found that he passed consistent stools of as large diameter as ever, which staggered his belief as to stricture.

I passed a large sized silver ball, and found a firm and fixed stop at six and a half inches, where it was evident the bowel was firmly attached to the sacrum. The examination conducted with care, gave no material pain. Not thinking it prudent to risk further disturbance of the parts at present, I directed a mild aperient, requesting to see him again in a fortnight.

Jan. 18. This gentleman visited me again, but I could neither get the smallest sized silver ball, nor a middle sized urethra bougie to pass further than six and a half inches, although the attempts were repeated with the greatest care; the necessity for which was intimated by a slight degree of pressure exciting a painful sense of heat in the fixed mass of the unyeilding disease. He now observed, that for the last two years he had occasionally been used to feel at the lower part of his loins a peculiar aching pain, most frequently when costive;, and also an occasional sense of heat in the bowel itself, similar to that he felt at present. Directed a gentle anodyne, as a night draught.

Feb. 2. Received another visit from my patient, who said he had derived comfort and relief from the medicine last ordered. He was anxious to have the application of the bougie repeated, but I thought it more prudent to postpone it, and consequently ordered his medicine to be continued.

Case 16.

Stricture in the Rectum.

Nov. 25. 1820. On calling at home, I found a gentleman waiting to see me, who had come from Bath, to desire my opinion. He stated that he had been attended by a surgeon in that city, who had told him he had a stricture in the rectum. He said he wished to know from me whether it was so or not. He had suffered no pain or uneasiness, direct or sympathetic. His bowels were somewhat variable, but tolerably regular; he said his principal' reason for doubting the existence of stricture, was his occasionally passing a solid stool of cousiderable diameter. On more close enquiring, however, it turned out, that the first portion only was large, the next being always squeezed and small; and that the length of the large mass never exceeded three or four inches.

In examination, the largest silver ball passed up to a stricture, which was not only a gradual contraction with progressively increased thickening of the parietes from the sphincter, but a disease firmly fixed in the pelvis. The ball wedged in, was with difficulty moved, when it had reached five inches. The intermediate space allowed the passage of the ball with some hesitation. The texture was evident, it was elastic and subcartilaginous. The introduction of a ball the next size smaller, gave precisely the same impression, only passing rather further into the contraction. The examination gave no pain, nor any sensation of uneasiness.

I stated it was most true that there was a stricture, not of a spasmodic, but permanent kind; and that the particular appearance of the fæces was owing to their having passed the stricture while soft, and having become hard in consistence, while retained in the lower part of the bowel.

He requested to know if I had any directions to give, with regard to his treatment; observing, that if possible, he would in two months see me again. I stated, that if a bougie could be passed beyond the stricture daily for a week or two, without pain, it appeared to me proper to proceed to the use of one a size larger; but that as to the particulars of the necessary treatment, or the particular tendency the complaint might manifest in future, they could only be ascertained by some continued attention to the effect of the means proposed.

Case 17.

Stricture in the Rectum.

June 13. 1820. I was consulted by a gentleman aged 78. He stated that about four years back he had a typhus fever, from which he recovered slowly; and that during his convalescence he first observed an irritation about the bladder, obliging him to void his urine more frequently than before. Independent of this, he thought that lately, although his bowels acted regularly, there was a defect in the power of expelling his fæces. He had already consulted several surgeons of eminence, one of whom, to satisfy himself there was no stricture in the urethra, had passed a bougie freely into the bladder. By the rectum, the finger at once ascertained that there was considerable enlargement of the prostate gland, but no apparent disease in the bowel. I therefore directed him for the evening a gentle anodyne, and for the morning an aperient draught requesting to see him again in a few days.

June 19. The bowels had been kept clear, and

he thought himself upon the whole rather better. I now examined the bowel with a bougie three-fourths of an inch in diameter, and at five inches found a firm stricture, not admitting the bougie; when the instrument was pushed half an inch further, the elasticity of the bowel brought it back again, proving it had not passed the disease, and also that the disease was not yet attached to the sacrum.

June 22. To day an elastic gum bougie half an inch in diameter was introduced, and passed with some resistance to six inches, where it became closely wedged into the stricture. In a few minutes the instrument was withdrawn. During the early part of July a bougie was several times introduced, and with evident benefit, the motions now passing with much more freedom than before. Being about to leave town, he was advised to continue the above plan of treatment.

Case 18.

Stricture in the Rectum.

Nov. 2. 1802. I was consulted by a gentleman, aged 51. who said he had a stricture in the rectum, which was frequently attended with much pain, and for which he had been under the care of various surgeons; some of whom had examined his complaint, and others not. To the extent that could be reached with the finger, the bowel was apparently sound; and elastic bougie half an inch in diameter traversed the first six inches freely, and then, with some hesitation passed through a part where the space was evidently diminished, and the surface irritable. For about an inch the progress of the instrument was impeded, after which it appeared to pass forward freely again. The examination gave no pain.

He had for the last ten years been subject to violent attacks of spasmodic diarrhœa, which returned every spring and fall; from these attacks he found no medicine relieve him till he tried opium, which invariably succeeded. He observed that in the early treatment of his stricture, a surgeon of great celebrity had put him to the most extreme distress and pain, by the manner in which he applied the bougie. One surgeon had recommended him to go to Leamington, and drink the waters; at which place he said, a medical gentleman had passed a bougie four inches, and told him he dare not pass it further, for at that part was a valve, which if injured would cost him his life. Under the direction of this gentleman he took calomel regularly for six weeks, with a very sore mouth most of the time. The only effect of this treatment, he thought, was to render him weaker and more irritable than before.

Nov. 5. The bougie introduced on the 2d inst. was now passed with more ease. He observed, he had for a long time been occasionally subject to an uneasiness and pain in his right hip, but never in the stricture itself.

Nov. 9. Had taken castor oil, which with straining had induced two small motions this morning. The instrument very gently introduced, would not pass beyond the sphincter. Suspecting displacement, I passed my finger, and found the whole of the diseased part accidentally brought within reach, so that the point of the finger evidently went through it into a relaxed and smooth part of the bowel. The extent of the disease was near two inches, its feel was that of an unequal thickening in the coats of the bowel, originating, as I conceived, in the cellular membrane, and not affecting the muscular fibres, for I found less actual contraction than I expected, the spaces between the thickened points admitting of relaxation.

Nov. 12. He believed he had taken cold, having some little frequency in passing water, with occasional chills, indisposition, and quickened pulse. He had taken ten grains of the compound powder of ipecacuan, in an evening draught for the last two days. Perspiration free over the body, but deficient in the legs and feet, which were always cold through the night. This morning castor oil operated easily. Rather more pain in the hip. Pulse 80; tongue clean.

Nov. 15. Thought himself in some respects rather better; but the bladder still irritable, with occasional darts of pain from behind forward into the glans: directed the volatile tincture of guaiacum, with tincture of opium in a draught to be taken twice a day. Passed an elastic gum bougie three fourths of an inch in diameter, eight inches along the rectum. It excited no uneasiness, and was therefore allowed to remain ten minutes.

Nov. 20. He said he was very poorly, and thought his complaints worse; for that he could get no motion without medicine, and when he felt the stool reach the seat of the stricture, he perceived a pain affecting the bladder with a desire to pass water, and until he had voided urine (which perhaps he could not do directly) he was unable to pass his stool, but afterwards he could. His features were shrunk, and he was evidently altering for the worse. Directing him an anodyne, I did not pass a bougie; but suspected some communication was about to form between the disease in the rectum, and the cavity of the bladder.

Nov. 28. Observed, that the sensations be occasionally felt in passing his water must, as he thought, depend on wind escaping from the bladder along the urethra, for that, sometimes a white mucous matter would make its appearance in little bubbles, accompanied with a noise as of air escaping from the orifice of the urethra. He said the idea had occurred to him doubtfully at first, but that he was now sure it must be so. The medicines were continued.

Dec. 7. This gentleman wrote to me, saying he was so poorly, that he should feel much obliged by my paying him a visit at his own house, at the east end of the town. I called the following day, and found him worse; complaining of severe and distressing spasms in various parts of his bowels.

A saline, ætherial and opiate draught was directed to be taken three or four times a day.

Dec. 11. Still in constant distress, from the severe and frequently returning spasms in the bowels. For his relief in aid of the former medicines, I now directed an opiate embrocation, to be rubbed upon the pit of the stomach during the continuance of spasm. From this application he derived much comfort and benefit.

Dec. 18. The spasms were still harrassing, but he had been also distressed by a pain in the right side, in the region of the liver; for this Mr. HEATH, who was his family surgeon, directed some leeches to be applied, a measure which soon relieved him. The spasms in the bowels, however, still continued to return, rendering his stomach irritable, his nights watchful, his days wearisome, and his prospects altogether hopeless. He continued to decline till Jan. 23. 1821, when he expired; worn away almost to a shadow, by great pain and long continued irritation.

On the second day after death, with the kind assistance of Mr. HEATH, I examined the body. The abdomen was much enlarged, but the body and limbs excessively emaciated. The bowels throughout were inflated, but were, generally speaking, sound; although a partial inflammatory blush upon the jejunum, pointed out the seat of the pain which had rendered it necessary to have recourse to the local abstraction of blood.

The stomach, partly contracted, was by no means diseased; neither was the pylorus materially thickened. The small intestines, except in being considerably enlarged, were healthy. The colon, although it had most probably being the seat of the spasmodic pains during life, exhibited no appearance to confirm the supposition. This bowel was equally and very considerably inflated through its whole course. The contents of the pelvis were removed, and washed, for more particular examination. On laying open the rectum, the extent of the principal disease was found to be confined to the extent of about two inches, the coats of the intestine being at this part much thickened, and diseased. The internal surface of the gut, for several inches above the stricture, exhibited several small spots, where ulceration of the mucous membrane had taken place; there was however no remaining appearance of surrounding inflammation.

In dissecting out the bowel, I found that an extensive abscess had formed in the cavity of the pelvis, upon the right side of the rectum; which abscess, it was afterwards ascertained, communicated with the gut. The stricture in the diseased part of the intestine was apparently the result of some very remote attack of inflammation, or if not, of some chronic excitement, inducing a secretion of a soft white matter, in tubercular masses, the mucous membrane of the bowel covering which, displayed the fine branches of several capillary arteries, shooting into the diseased structure.

The abscess, into which it appeared some previously deposited masses of coagulable lymph had been let loose by the ulcerative process, was situated, as abovementioned, on the right side of the intestine; near the seat of those dull heavy pains which so long had affected the hip.

In the bladder, directly behind the prostate gland, was a membranous fold, similar in situation, and somewhat similar in appearance, to that described and engraved in the history of a case related elsewhere.* In the present case, however, this membranous fold did not project forward enough to produce the serious consequence which, in the former instance, proved fatal; but it was highly vascular, irritable, and upon its margin fungated. Raising the divided edges of the bladder at this part, lifted up this preternatural valve, exposing a large ulcerated opening, by which a full-sized urethra bougie passed at once from the bladder, through the abscess, into the thickened and diseased part of the rectum.

CASE 19.

Stricture in the Rectum.

Feb. 18. 1821. I was consulted by a gentleman, about thirty-five years of age, from the neighbourhood of Manchester, who said his com-

* Practical observations on the diseases of the Urinary Organs.

plaints, for which he had consulted many medical gentlemen, were rather peculiar. Some had supposed one thing, and some another. Several had been led to think the liver affected; and one of the last physicians he had consulted had stated his conviction that the mesenteric glands were enlarged. His principal uneasiness, he said, was about the lower part of the belly, where, especially after fatigue, he experienced a sense of irksome weight, and continuing uneasiness. His complaints were of long standing; and fifteen or twenty years back, when in their commencement, he used to feel occasional pain just behind the left hip, affecting the whole limb, which had become permanently weakened, and perceptibly emaciated. His bowels were somewhat variable, but generally regular, and very easily acted upon by purgatives. The stools, when solid, were of large diameter.

I stated to him that from the account he had given me, I was clearly of opinion that his bowels were out of health; and that as I could neither perceive enlargement or tenderness, either in the region of the liver, or any other part of the abdomen, I was inclined to think the principal complaint was in the bowels; which complaint, by a steady perseverance in the use of proper medicines, might perhaps in time be removed; but that I should consider it right to ascertain by examination, whether the rectum was in a healthy state. This he said was a measure that not one of his numerous medical attendants had ever thought of, but that he should of course submit to whatever was judged necessary. I directed an infusion of gentian and cascarilla.

Feb. 20. Said the medicines had perfectly agreed with him, and that he was himself of opinion that his principal complaints were in the bowels, because he uniformly found that when he took a hearty meal, he felt the weight and uneasiness come on, and that as the digestive process went forward, he became progressively easier and lighter. His bowels were not in a favourable state for examination, being rather confined. Directed the decoction of bark, with infusion of cascarilla.

Feb. 23. Observed that he was somewhat better, his bowels being relaxed. I therefore examined the rectum, passing a ball seven eighths of an inch diameter, with some little constriction, at three inches on to five inches, where it stopped short in a gradual contraction of the bowel, which was thickened, and partially attached to the sacrum. On repeating the examination with a ball of three eighths of an inch, it passed easily on to five and a half inches; but no art could get it further.

I was now able to state to him, not only the truth, but the whole truth, acquainting him that his complaint was a stricture of the rectum, that it might and would require the occasional and judicious use of instruments as well as the employment of proper medicines. In answer to his enquiries relating to the affection of his left leg and thigh, he was acquainted that, provided the primary complaint, which was seated in the bowel, was gradually relieved by the treatment, of which

I had little doubt, the affection of the limb, nervous and sympathetic, would be relieved also.

Case 20.

Scirrhous Stricture in the Rectum.

A labouring man, aged fifty-two, with much pain in the loins, became subject to irritation at the neck of the bladder. The urine flowed freely, but was followed by pain and straining, which in a few weeks became very violent. His bowels were confined, so as frequently to require physic. After three months he applied to St. George's Infirmary, and I was requested to see him, in February, 1810. He had then severe pains in the back and loins, with lameness of one thigh. There was no appearance of ill health about the limb, but as the bowels were costive, some opening medicine was directed.

The distress in making water increased the urine depositing a thick white sediment. The irritation in the bladder allowed him no rest, frequently inducing irresistible desire, though with fruitless efforts to pass a motion. Bougies passed into the urethra threw no light upon the case; I therefore examined by the rectum, which was firmly contracted just within reach of the finger.

Extreme irritability rendering the common bougie objectionable, a curved wax taper was introduced, and allowed to remain half an hour;

and after some days, the operation was repeated. The wax bougie was then exchanged for one of tallow: this proved to be the only tolerable mode of operating by pressure. To the finger, the inner membrane of the bowel felt as if puckered up into small short ridges, or folds; the other coats of the intestine were evidently much thickened, as well as contracted. The disease was firmly attached to the sacrum.

He soon became subject to severe spasmodic darting pains in the strictured part, all the symptoms gaining ground, till any further attempt at relief by the use of the bougie was given up. Worn down by extreme irritation and pain with dropsical effusion into the abdomen, he sunk and died, April 10. 1810.

On opening the body, a very extensive scirrhous disease was found in the omentum and stomach; but the largest mass was formed by the rectum. At the upper part of the pelvis this intestine was firmly fixed to the spine and sacrum, by an extensive thickening of parts around the gut, the coats of which had undergone a very complete conversion into the true scirrhous structure.

Removed from the pelvis, the anterior line of the intestine was laid open, from the anus upwards, dividing through the stricture. The contraction had commenced several inches above the sphincter, extending thence upwards and downwards. The section of the disease, from the margin of the villous coat to that of the peritoneal covering, measured three quarters of an inch in thickness.

STRICTURE.

The urinary bladder, in structure undiseased, was exceedingly contracted, and consequently thickened, the effect of long-continued irritation, from sympathy. The cavity would scarcely contain a table-spoonful; the inner membrane was exceedingly vascular.*

Case 21.

Inflammation of the Colon, terminating in Effusion.

The subject of the following case was a lady, whose complaints had, by various practitioners, been attributed to disease in the liver; upon which presumption she had, in the early part of her illness, been repeatedly subjected to the influence of mercury, without benefit. Of several who had seen and attended her, Dr. Hooper was the only physician who could never be persuaded to believe her complaints hepatic, notwithstanding constant local uneasiness, frequently severe pain, and a degree of tumour below the cartilages of the ribs on the right side, with occasional pain at the shoulder. The action of the bowels was irregular: sometimes there were twenty-four stools in as many hours; at others, strong purgatives were required to be frequently given for days together, without effect.

* A coloured engraving of the appearance of the bladder is given in my observations on the diseases of the Urinary Organs.

A variety of medicines were directed; but opiates only, when powerful, gave much relief. In the latter period of her illness, I was desired to see her on account of dropsy. She went through the operation of tapping four times, and on each of these occasions I drew off, on the average, four gallons of fluid. She died Feb. 12. 1820.

On examination, I found a thickened, discoloured, soft and elastic tumour lying across the upper part of the abdomen, a circumscribed portion of which tumour had visibly raised the external parietes, previous to their being laid aside. From the right extremity of this tumour several strong adhesions passed off to the adjacent surface of the parietes; from its anterior part also several short thick cords, the result of effusion, were firmly attached to the peritoneum, just within the scrobiculus cordis. The tumour itself turned out to be the stomach and transverse arch of the colon, closely and completely adherent to each other; the former viscus much discoloured, the latter much diseased, so altered in texture, and so much thickened, as to have entirely lost its natural characters.

The tumour, which during life had given an additional cast of ambiguity to the case, proved to be merely a part of the stomach, which, from the adhesions by which at most other points it was confined, had occasionally formed a tender, irritable, and painful point, externally.

The adhesions just mentioned were exceedingly strong, and all proceeded from the colon, which had evidently been the seat of the primary inflammation. The bands attached to the scrobiculus cordis clearly explained the distressing sense of gnawing, or burning, or glowing heat, with the occasional sense of pulling, or drawing at that part from which she was never altogether free.

The ascites proved to have been merely the consequence of the derangement in the function of absorption, resulting from the first inflammation; for the liver was healthy in structure, although its peritoneal covering was somewhat thickening.

Case 22.

*Inflammation in the Colon, followed by stricture.**

For as many as seven or eight years before his death, the Rev. Dr. M—y had usually about twenty purging stools in the course of the twenty-four hours, from a complaint in his bowels, which he believed originated in a blow previously received upon the side of the belly. The principal seat of this complaint he always pointed out so exactly in his emaciated state, that it was observed at the time it must be in the colon, where it passes down on the outside of the left kidney. It was thought probable there might be some contraction or ulceration at that place.

* Extracted from the MS. in Mr. HEAVISIDE's museum, where the diseased parts are preserved.

About three years before his death he had a fistula in ano, for which he was successfully cut, and, from the time of the inflammation that led to the fistula, he was sensible that the lower part of the rectum remained in an awkward uneasy state, rendering it painful and difficult to introduce the tube, in giving an injection.

Subsequent to this period his medical friends were of opinion that no more could be done than to palliate, and procure sleep. He was directed to have recourse to opiates, and was at times, by these means, much refreshed and comforted. He latterly became exceedingly emaciated, from the ill state of his heatlh, added to close application to the duties of his profession, which, notwithstanding pain and sickness, he never willingly neglected. Before he died, his legs became dropsical, and swelled very much.

On examining the body, the opinion formed of the disorder proved to be correct. The small intestines were healthy; the cœcum, and beginning of the colon, much inflated, but not imflamed. The transverse arch of the colon was also much inflated, but it had likewise the appearance of inflammation. The distended part of the colon terminated opposite the lower end of the left kidney, where there was an annular stricture of the gut. At this part the contracted intestine had the feel of firm flesh, and had evidently suffered previous inflammation. The diseased intestine being slit up, was internally inflamed, and superficially ulcerated, paticularly towards the seat of the stricture. At the stricture the passage was very small, winding irregularly through an inch and a half of compact but ulcerated substance. Below this where the colon passes over the psoas and illiac vessels, it was in its natural state. The rectum had suffered much from disease, and, for a finger's length to within two inches of the anus, was contracted almost to the size of a goose-quill, and of a livid colour. The lower two inches of the rectum were not so much contracted, but of the same livid colour. The inner surface of this part of the gut was traversed by many short flattened bands, somewhat resembling the fasciculated structure within the heart. This latter appearance was the effect, no doubt, of inflammation, at the time when the abscess formed, near the side of the gut.

CHAPTER II.

ON ULCERATION OF THE INTERNAL SURFACE OF THE INTESTINE.

SECT. I.

On the Causes of the Disease.

63. THE variety of effects produced by sympathetic complaints, and the irregularity of symptoms, frequently make it difficult to ascertain the causes of disease. We know that inflammation so generally precedes ulceration, that we are naturally led to conclude these two actions necessarily connected together, as cause and effect, and that the latter must be invariably preceded by the former. The certainty of this point, however, may, I think, be doubted.

64. In some late researches into the minute appearances of disease in the bones*, I have unquestionably detected absorption, or in other words ulceration, unconnected with any character of preceding inflammation; and in the dissection of those who have died from disease in the alimentary canal, I have in various instances found so little

---

* Published in the Transactions of the Medico-Chirurgical Society.

trace of inflammatory action around spots of apparently recent ulceration, that I cannot help doubting whether, under some circumstances, irritation in the bowels may not establish a degree of excitement sufficient to induce ulceration, without any distinct appearance of inflammatory action.

65. In considering the occasional causes of irritation in the bowels, it has often appeared to me that the functions of the liver, and consequently the properties of the bile, are very much influenced by external circumstances; and that those who are but little exposed to the inclemency of weather, are nevertheless liable to suffer from an acrimony in the bilious secretion, as a consequence of common cold, an effect quite distinct from the increased quantity of thin mucous fluid excreted from the bowels in dysenteric diarrhœa; the first exciting a distressing sense of heat, and even excoriation about the anus; the second passing off without any such irritation, although they are both occasionally attended with an irksome sense of weight, and bearing down in the rectum. These observations, which I have very repeatedly had the opportunity of making when abroad with the army, have lately been set in a correct though conspicuous point of view, in the valuable works of Dr. Johnson, on Atmospherical Influence, and particularly on the Diseases of Tropical Climates.

66. A very painfully irritable state of the rectum is sometimes caused by disease in some neighbouring part, particularly the womb. Irritation from this cause will require peculiar treatment.

67. The functions of the alimentary canal may be permanently deranged, marking a sort of intermediate state between health and disease, if possible, more important than disease itself; for if treated with that early attention its cousequence demands, it almost invariably admits of being set right, while many of the eventual diseases of these viscera are of very uncertain event, under the best treatment.

68. When the intestines possess a permanent excess of irritability, they will require attentive and patient management. Extremely prone to constant relaxation, and frequently to spasm also, there will be great difficulty in bringing them back to the quiet steady performance of their healthy functions. This intermediate state I have so frequently seen pave the way to actual disease, that I am persuaded there are very few diseases of the bowels that are not occasionally brought on by its continued influence.*

69. It seems probable that this state of permanently increased irritability, and the particular complaints to which it gives rise, is frequently allied to a local scorbutic diathesis; it is of importance to determine this point correctly, for if there is such tendency, nothing is more formidable in its ultimate results, nor any thing more easily removed, by early and proper attention. This opinion is rendered probable by the nature and tendency of the symptoms which, during life, I have frequently watched and considered; but is especially confirmed

---

* Cases 23. and 24.

by the appearance after death, and particularly by the rapidity with which putrefaction sometimes takes place. The latter circumstance is well illustrated by an observation made by Dr. HUXHAM, who mentions a disease in the colon, which appears to me to have been the consequence of continued inattention to diet on the one hand, and, continued neglect of medical advice on the other. The patient was of a bilious scorbutic habit, subject to flatulence and cholic pains. These appear to have been unattended to, and he subsequently had tenesmus, and frequent bilious, purulent and fœtid stools, occasionally with blood; arising from the neglect of the former admonitory disorders. The latter complaints, as might be expected, were not to be removed. His appetite unsteady the action of his bowels always uneven, he languished out only two years of misery, having taken a great variety of medicines in vain, nothing but laudanum affording him even temporary relief. On examining the parts after death, the ileum was found in one part inflamed from irritation, while the colon was in a gangrenous state, and the internal surface of the rectum as black as ink, from complete mortification. The head of the colon had formed, through the medium of adhesion, an ulcerated opening into the rectum, by which most of the contents of the bowels were supposed latterly to have passed. But, although the patient had been troubled with a looseness before his death, the greater part of the colon was stuffed up with indurated fæces; the liquid parts of the fecal matter having passed directly into the rectum through the ulcerated orifice, while the more solid parts were retained in the colon.* Another instance, somewhat similar, will be noticed presently. (88.)

70. Inflammation alone may produce ulceration in the mucous membrane of the bowels, but I have most commonly observed this change occur where inflammatory action has evidently operated in connection with irritation, from the presence of acrimonious matter in the intestines. In one instance I have found irritation from the long-continued passage of the urine through a fictitious opening in the rectum, in a case of diseased urethra and prostate gland, produce ulceration of the bowel, inducing a very irksome and distressing tenesmus, from which the patient could never be effectually relieved.

71. External violence may sometimes induce ulceration of the bowels, but provided the bruise as been moderate in degree, and that the intestine is not absolutely lacerated, the internal surface may separate by sloughing, and do perfectly well.†

Sect. 2.

On the Symptoms and Appearances of the Disease.

72. ULCERATION in the bowels will, in its commencement, generally be connected with pain in

---

* Phil. Trans. vol. xxxvii. † Case 31.

some part of the abdominal region, usually acute, and more or less intense, dependent on the turn of constitution favouring either phlegmonous or erysipelatous action.

73. Obstinate costiveness, extreme tenderness or severe pain in the belly, heat of skin, thirst, and white tongue, hard and quick pulse, will sometimes lead to a suspicion of acute inflammation, requiring diligent attention, and the most active treatment; while in other cases, with heat of skin, thirst, foul tongue, and local pain, the pulse, although quickened, will not be remarkably hard.

74. Where, consequent to some of the above signs of inflammation, ulceration follows, it will be either circumscribed or diffused. When this process is circumscribed, I think the danger greatest, for in these cases principally I have found the ulcer penetrate through the muscular and external coats of the intestine, an event almost uniformly fatal. Where, on the other hand, the ulceration is diffused over a surface of considerable extent, the intensity of the preceding inflammation may be presumed to have been less, at least I have in various instances found a great extent of bowel thus affected, without its having penetrated beyond the internal or mucous membrane of the gut.

75. Should ulceration make its way quickly through all the coats of the bowel, the escape of its contents into the general cavity of the abdomen immediately follows; an event productive of the most distressing pain, and extreme tenderness of the belly. with increase of fever, from peritoneal

inflammation, which, under these circumstances, is, I believe, invariably fatal.

76. In some cases, inflammation affects all the coats of the bowel at the same time, and adhesion becomes the means of saving the life of the patient.

77. When effusion happens in this way, coagulable lymph is poured out upon the bowel, producing adhesion, either to the external parietes of the abdomen, or, perhaps, to some other part of the intestinal tube, by which medium the ulcerative action making its way through the mass of lymph, producing an outlet for the contained matters through the external integuments, or effects a passage out of one into another part of the intestinal canal; in either case preventing the mischief that would arise from the contents of the bowels escaping into the general cavity of the belly. Occasionally the adhesive process puts an entire stop to the further progress of mischief. The symptoms and appearances connected with this tendency are strongly illustrated by the 86th case, in the Surgical Observations.

78. An instance, showing that the process of adhesion, through a salutary effort of nature, is not always to be depended upon, may be found in an interesting case, were it may be taken for granted there had been ulceration of the mucus membrane of the colon, although in examination after death no remaining trace of inflammation appeared. It is related by Dr. STOKER, in the Transactions of the Irish College of Physicians. In this instance irritation from the perpetual load

of contents had brought on ulceration; although the accidental bursting of the weakest part of the over-distended bowel proved the immediate cause of death.

79. Provided the ulceration is merely superficial, every thing may go on favourably, and end well. The constitutional symptoms, under proper treatment, giving way, the ulcerated parts may become clean, and assume healthy actions; suppuration be succeeded by cicatrization, and as the extent of exposed surface diminishes, the strength will increase, the constitutional sympathy evinced by the foul tongue, heat of skin, and disturbed pulse, will decrease, and at length entirely vanish.

80. The preceding observations more immediately regard primary affections of the bowels; but it is of equal importance, in a practical point of view, to recollect that the intestinal canal is sometimes affected secondarily, under circumstances which nevertheless may concern the safety as well as comfort of the patient. Inflammation may come on, and abscess follow in some part of the abdomen, attended with fever, local tumour, and pain; where every thing will depend no less upon the watchfulness than the discernment of the practitioner.

81. The probability of matter having formed must be judged of by the diminished hardness of the pulse, and the decline of the other feverish symptoms; by the cool and relaxed skin, the decrease of local pain, and generally, also, by the occurrence of rigors, or chilliness. The favour-

able view here is the hope that the abscess may, through the medium of adhesion, attach itself to some part of the bowels, and in this way find an outlet consistent with the safety of the patient. In this event, the ulcerated opening in the bowel, abstractedly, is of no real importance, it merely allows the escape of matter, as long as necessary; when the abscess has contracted and closed, it readily heals up.*

82. The appearance of blood in the stools, independent of piles, has been held to be a criterion of ulceration in the bowels. Upon this evidence, however, I place no reliance. It is true, that in dysenteric complaints, when the urgency and straining to pass a motion is perpetual or violent, blood is frequently voided, and it is reasonable to believe it proceeds from the ulcerated parts of the bowels, where these are low down; but ulceration frequently exists in the superior parts of the great intestine, where these irksome symptoms can have little influence; and this circumstance may explain why in some cases the stools have never been tinged with blood, notwithstanding ulceration of the mucous membrane of the bowels has been found to exist after death.

In point of fact, the motions being free from blood is no proof that the bowels are free from ulceration; neither does the presence of blood in the stools prove ulceration to have taken place.

83. I have in several instances attended persons

* Case 28.

attacked with severe pains and relaxation in the bowels, the evacuations having more or less the appearance of pure blood; in two of these cases the same kind of matter was repeatedly rejected by vomiting. The attack has continued some time, the fluids passed sometimes resembling thick, dark, bilious stools, at others appearing like grumous unhealthy blood. In these complaints, the fits of griping pain have occurred after the manner of spasm, being presently succeeded by a free evacuation, from which the patient has experienced temporary relief. The quantity of this fluid matter passed at one time has been frequently equal to one, two, or even three pints.

84. The real nature of this disorder has been hitherto but little investigated. In one case, however, in which a second attack terminated fatally, with permission of the physician who had attended, I availed myself of the opportunity for ascertaining the seat and cause of the hæmorrhage, and I think of the disease also. The bleeding had taken place from the capillary or exhalent arteries upon the internal surface of the great intestine, and although it was evident that every part of the bowel had been a bleeding surface, no part had suffered ulceration, nor was any part inflamed, though the whole was very red.*

On comparing the symptoms that attended in the above case with what I had previously seen of a similar kind, I was convinced that this disorder is a

* Practical Observations in Surgery, Case 83.

consequence of a particular stage of the scorbutic diathesis; although it is not always attended with the spongy state of gums, which is one of the strongest general characters of that disease. Taking it upon this ground, I have since been enabled to succeed in curing the complaint. The opinion that the fluid usually voided in this disorder is principally blood, was that of an eminent and excellent professor of the Edinburgh school.*

85. M. PORTAL has published upon this subject an excellent memoir, which I have lately read with much pleasure and profit. He states that the black matter evacuated is not bile, but blood, having no trace of bitterness, not dissolving, like bile in cold water, nor giving any green colour to the water; but that it is pure blood, which in the bodies of those examined after death may be seen to transude from the blood-vessels of the stomach, and small, not large intestines. His words are " dans les intestins greles et non gros." This exception, however, is an error that any one might readily have fallen into, arising merely from his having seen the disease affect the small, but not the large intestines.

86. The disease is considered to be the consequence of a local plethora of liver, spleen, or some other viscus, creating plethora in the corresponding arteries, and exudation in consequence; the black colour of the arterial blood arising from its meeting with carbonic acid gas in the general

* Dr. HOME. Clinical Experiments.

canal. The cramp and spasm of the stomach and bowels, sometimes caused by violent affections of mind, are considered capable of giving rise to this complaint. It is admitted sometimes to depend on the scorbutic diathesis, being then produced either by the over-loaded state of the liver and spleen, or by the altered condition of the blood, peculiar to scurvy.

When produced by plethora, bleeding by leeches from the hæmorrhoidal veins; in other cases the use of acids, wine, and tonics, are recommended.*

87. Regarding the history and treatment of malæna, M. RODAMEL has related a highly instructive case, in which blood first passed from the stomach by vomiting, and then downwards into the bowels, creating increasing distension, constant distress, with failing irregular pulse, and cold sweats, the bowels obstinately refusing all impression from purging and injections; the mechanical irritation of the rectum, by the introduction of a large gum catheter its whole length, was followed by the evacuation of three large pot-fuls of matter, black and bilious; the abdomen was thus unloaded, and the patient to all appearance expiring, gradually revived, and eventually recovered.

The same thing happened a second time, and was relieved by the same means.

The disease was believed to be connected with the putrescent diathesis.†

* Memoires de la Société Medicale d'Emulation, tom. ii.
† Mem. de la Soc. Med. d'Emulation, tom. vi.

88. A very interesting case has been given by Mr. HILL, which appears to me to have been originally a bleeding from the villous coat of the bowels, which, after a long course of severe and varied sufferings, proved fatal; but not till it had reduced the diseased viscera to that condition that at the time of death nearly the whole of the rectum had actually mortified; the fragments of an extensive portion of the bowel, and the fæcal contents, being found loose in the cavity of the pelvis.*

The quantity of blood that has in some instances been thrown off from the stomach is astonishing. A case is recorded where the enormous quantity of twelve pounds and upwards were vomited up in the space of two hours, and the patient perfectly recovered.†

89. The appearances that occur upon dissection, in ulcerated bowels, will vary. In the early progress, the blush of increased vascularity will be more extensive, but as certain points of intense action become established, the excitement upon the intermediate space declines, till at length ulceration takes place. When the cellular membrane is once exposed, it may fall into a sloughy state, from the debility incident to previous excess of action, or from the presence of acrimonious matters in the bowels, now brought into immediate contact with it. Should the constitutional health be good, this may not occur; healthy suppuration may take place, and the excitement being moderate,

---

* Edin. Med. Journ. vol. xii.   † Phil. Trans. vol. xxxvii.

a granulating surface forms, soon beginning to heal over, and eventually covered with a cicatrix of a fine smooth texture.

90. The new surface thus produced is not to be supposed in all respects equal to the original structure. On the contrary, it is destitute of the power of absorption, one of the functions of the natural mucous membrane; it is also found to resemble other newly formed parts, in being more irritable than the original surface of the intestines. From these two circumstances are derived the only permanent inconveniences I know of, resulting from ulceration in the bowels, where the complaint ends favourably; and they generally escape observation, unless where the disease has been severe. Where, however, a large extent of intestine has been so affected, I have found that the diminished quantity of support derived to the system by absorption, and the constant tendency to diarrhœa from the extreme irritability, have arrested the progress of recovery after the ulcerated parts had healed, and have subsequently proved fatal, in spite of every effort that I could make to counteract their influence. A striking and singular demonstation of these interesting and curious facts has been already brought forward.*

---

* Practical Observations in Surgery, Case 77.

Sect. 3.

On the Treatment.

61. THE symptoms that lead to a suspicion of inflammatory action in the bowels, ought in every instance to be watched with the closest attention; for it frequently happens, that pains, at first occasional and spasmodic, will very quickly take on the more permanent and serious characters of inflammation.

92. The medical treatment of inflammation must be directed entirely by circumstances (34.). The continued exhibition of mild aperients, in divided doses, will in these complaints frequently operate well by passing through the bowels, although at first they may have been rejected by vomiting. The combination of the neutral salines with the infusion and tincture of senna, are, I think, in general less apt to produce sickness than castor oil, but it will be often necessary to try a variety of medicines before any succeed. With a view to moderate arterial action, it may be also expedient to direct, at intervals, some of the saline diaphoretics. A large and gently laxative enema, if ordered to be carefully and slowly injected, will sometimes by its volume, as well as warmth, assist essentially in promoting salutary relaxation of the bowels.

93. If the patient be young, and the symptoms strongly marked, with much pain and local tender-

ness, the practitioner will require all his discernment in determining the moment for having recourse to the lancet and warm bath. The benefit to be derived from the former means is well known, and the powerful influence of the latter is sometimes very great. I recollect trying it once to the fullest extent, in the hospital of the 82d regiment. A boy had a most obstinate attack of inflammation on the lungs, resisting very large and repeated bleeding, blistering, and every other means usually employed. The oppression and severe pain in the chest remaining unabated, and the pulse failing so as to render the further abstraction of blood positively unsafe, I determined that at least he should not die of the disease, if I could help it; and therefore directed the hospital sergeant to set him in a warm bath, and keep him there till he fainted away; then to lift him out and lay him between warm blankets till he revived, when he was to be again immersed in the bath till he fainted a second time. He was directed to continue these successive operations until the boy felt relief in the chest. The experiment succeeded completely; after several immersions the complaint gave way, and the young man recovered perfectly.

94. A very essential, if not the most important point, consists in establishing a free and relaxed state of the bowels. Till this point is achieved, the patient cannot be considered safe; but this once effected, and febrile action somewhat relieved, the case will, or at least ought, to end well, with the assistance of proper saline or antimo-

nial diaphoretics, and due attention to diet, which during the season of convalescence, should be of the lightest possible description.

Where the evidence of inflammatory action is doubtful, and the affection is discovered on examination to be produced by disease in the neighbourhood, the object must be to soothe, quiet, and compose the part, by an anodyne treatment.*

95. Where the symptoms indicate a tendency to erysipelatous action, the abstraction of blood must be directed with caution, the dependence being rather upon diaphoretics and opiates, in small doses, taking great care at the same time to ensure regular action of the bowels, by the occasional use of gentle aperients.

By these means ill consequences may generally be prevented, the inflammation being subdued without allowing time for the establishment of serious mischief; sometimes, however, it happens otherwise, and ulceration may then ensue.

96. It has been observed, that where ulceration is confined to the mucous membrane, the complaint may be frequently relieved and cured, provided the real nature of the case is known, and the treatment adapted to the state of constitution, as well as to the local affection. That ulceration, when it extends through all the coats of a bowel, must be almost invariably fatal, is proved by the appearances and symptoms in Cases 78. and 79., in the Surgical Observations.

* Cases 25, 26, and 27.

97. The probability of ulceration having made its way through all the coats of the intestine, must be calculated from the duration and degree of the early symptoms, contrasted with those that may subsequently arise, from a sudden attack of peritoneal inflammation, without any obvious external cause. Under such circumstances, every exertion should be made to keep down arterial action, by blood-letting general and local, and by every other means. The possibility of this event, in any case of ulcerated bowels, will point out the necessity for keeping a watchful eye upon the progress of the disease, without exciting unnecessary alarm in the minds of the family; yet with care that the moment new symptoms arise their probable importance may be so appreciated by the friends of the patient, as not to subject either the discernment or the conduct of the practitioner to unmerited censure.

98. Where there is reason to believe ulcerationof the mucous membrane of the bowels has taken place, the most minute attention must be paid to diet, and to every circumstance that can, in any way, influence that curative process, the accomplishment of which rests with the powers of the constitution.

99. A principal object will be to prevent the formation of any acrimonious matter in the bowels, taking care to preserve an easy and regular transmission of their contents. We must observe with attention, through the pulse and tongue, the ever-varying state of the system, and either raise it carefully when prone to depres-

sion, or cautiously moderate any tendency to excess of tone; thus endeavouring to maintain that quietude of balance most conducive to eventual recovery.

100. These observations are the result of expericuce, and not of reading. I have constantly found that were ulceration in the bowels has once taken place, the least irregularity in diet, the most trifling derangement of stomach, will excite uneasiness, or pain, in the seat of the complaint, generally followed by a tendency to diarrhœa; and in those cases where, from the ulcer being low down, it could sometimes be partially seen, the nature and cause of these symptoms have been proved by the unfavourable change manifested in the appearance of the ulcerated surface.

101. The indications to be held in view may be occasionally forwarded by the use of mild diaphoretics, but will generally be fulfilled most advantageously by the exhibition of light tonics, combined either with aromatics or opiates. In cases of this description, Dr. HOOPER is occasionally in the habit of directing various light combinations of steel; and in some instances that I have seen with astonishing advantage. The effect of any of these means must of course be occasionally regulated either by castor oil, or some other aperient.

102. Where an ulcer is sufficiently low down to be within reach in any examination per anum, it has been supposed that the disposition of the diseased surface may be improved by the injection of astringent fluids into the rectum. Upon any

treatment conducted on this principle I should not place much reliance. Not that I have frequently found it fail, having little experience of the effect of local applications under these circumstances; but well knowing, the habits and structure of all parts of the alimentary canal are very much the same, I am persuaded that the most useful, and in general the only successful, efforts to remove or to relieve the disease, must be made through the medium of the constitution; taking care to prevent the occurrence of local irritation, as already stated.

Where the ulceration has been confined to the sphincter of the anus, I have, in one instance, derived advantage from the application of a solution of the argentum nitratum.*

103. When an ulcer in the bowels proceeds from an abscess in the neighbourhood, the treatment must be directed to the abscess alone, the ulcerated opening from it being of no comparative importance. In this case, the first attention must be paid to the employment of all the usual modes of depletion, while there is any chance of preventing the more serious consequences of inflammation; when these fail, fomentations and poultice will generally succeed in bringing the abscess forward; and when the contents have made their way into the bowels, the copious discharge of blood and pus will sufficiently explain the state of the case, and according to circumstances in-

* Case 30.

dicate the propriety of baving recourse to tonic medicines, and strengthening diet, or the contrary.*

104. The occurrence of large discharges, apparently of blood from the bowels, is generally unconnected with ulceration; and as this particular disorder of the intestinal canal has been but little adverted to, though always serious, and often fatal; I may be excused in making some few practical remarks regarding this kind of hæmorrhage.

105. In July, 1811, I visited a gentleman, who towards the decline of life was attacked with this disorder. Owing to various circumstances he had long experienced a declension both in health and spirits; when he was suddenly seized with a severe vomiting and purging, which, from the appearance of the stools, seemed at first to resemble cholera morbus. There were frequent spasmodic pains in the bowels, a small weak pulse, and extreme prostration of strength. The execssive debility, and the severity of the pains were such, that when the spasms came on, the accumulated contents of the rectum passed at once away, without any power of restraint. On the third day the vomiting declined, but the stools, although less copious, were now evidently blood, little, if at all, changed by mixture with other fluids. Mr. HEAVISIDE, who was the surgeon in attendance, had little hope of his recovery; but assisted by medicine, and a light nutritious diet, he was eventually, though very slowly, restored to health.

* Case 28.

The next case of which I had the opportunity of seeing not only the progress, but also the termination, I have formerly adverted to (84.); it was one that I could only view in the light of a scorbutic complaint. Upon several accounts this case excited my particular attention.

106. In January, 1817, I had again an opportunity of seeing the disease, being consulted by a man aged forty, who for several months had passed almost daily, blood by the rectum, without my being able to trace any disease in the anus, or in the bowel above it. He some days voided a dessert spoonful, at others half a pint. It generally passed alone, but sometimes with fæces. This case was marked by spongy, but not bleeding gums; but it agreed with the others in extreme constitutional debility, and excessive depression of spirits, and might be clearly traced to a preceding course of low, poor, salted diet. I directed him to eat fresh food and vegetables, and ordered him to take also the juice of four lemons every day, in lemonade, or otherwise. In a fortnight his complaints were better, but the plan was now changed for astringents. The sulphuric acid, tincture of kino, rectified spirit of turpentine, and various aluminous mixtures, were tried in succesion, but without success; they produced severe spasmodic pains, costiveness, and sickness at stomach, without in the least checking the hæmorrhage. These medicines laid aside, he was again ordered the lemon-juice, with the addition of bark and aromatics, the bowels being kept in a state of regu-

larity by castor-oil. Under this treatment his complaints gave way, and by two months' perseverance he found himself entirely recovered; his spirits and strength being essentially improved, and the appearance of blood in his stools quite removed.

107. Where ulcers in the bowels have healed, I have observed (90.) that the new surface is neither capable of absorbing nor of bearing irritation, so well as the original structure. The first of these peculiarities is only felt as an inconvenience where the ulceration has been extensive, but the second is often extremely distressing. The least change in diet, the least degree of cold, will bring on a sudden attack of looseness, with griping pains in the bowels, subjecting the patient to weakness, and temporary exhaustion.

108. Under these circumstances I have found no means of relief comparable to opium, judiciously adminstered. I say judiciously, because its power of regulating this particular disposition is entirely dependent upon its proper direction, and careful management; if carelessly exhibited, it will presently become so necessary to the patient, that it cannot be laid aside, and it may then be doubted whether the remedy may not prove worse than the disease.

109. Attention should also be paid to the clothing. The habit of constantly wearing flannel next the skin cannot be too strongly recommended, especially in this variable climate. It tends to encourage the insensible perspiration, and renders

the patient infinitely less liable to cold from sudden alteration of temperature.

Case 23.

Deranged Action of Bowels.

Dec. 21. 1820. A gentleman called to consult me, whose complaints related to the habitual state of his bowels, discomposed by the slightest cause, generally too relaxed, sometimes violently so; with occasional pain, but more frequently uneasiness, and flatulent tension. He said he had been in the East Indies, where he had liver complaints, and used a great deal of mercury, which ran so violently off by the bowels, that he had never been able to bear mercurial medicines since. Two things he observed he was quite sure of; the one, that he had no complaint now that related to the liver; the other, that there was no affection in the way of stricture in the rectum; for that a surgeon of eminence, by whom he had been attended several months, had passed a bougie to satisfy his mind upon this point.

I told him that medicine might render him very material assistance, but that a careful attention to his diet and general habits might do even more than medicine; that there was little doubt on my mind that he might in time perfectly recover his health, but that experience had taught me that the treatment of cases of this nature required more patience and perseverance than many persons possessed, and that for this reason alone they were frequently deemed incurable.

I thought it right to direct him two or three grains of the pil. hydrarg. to take at night, and a very gentle aperient the following morning, as a preliminary measure, requesting to see him again in a few days.

Upon his second visit he acquainted me, that although he had felt a dread of the pill, he had taken it, and, as I had previously assured him, he had found it operate very mildly. I told him, the object must now be to attend constantly to his bowels, observing so to regulate his diet, as to avoid creating disturbance in the bowels, and taking at the same time such medicines as, by imperceptible degrees, might operate, by restoring them to their original tone and strength; for that in proportion as their natural powers increased, irritability, and the symptoms arising from it would diminish, and at last disappear.

Understanding he intended returning into the country, I prescribed for him a light tonic, to be taken every morning; pointing out this as the first step towards his improvement.

CASE 24.

Deranged action of Bowels.

Dec. 23. 1820. I was consulted by a middle-aged gentleman, for a complaint that was productive of constant vexation and distress. A continual tendency to diarrhœa, much aggravated by taking any acid, fresh fruit, or other things that were apt to disagree with him. Three years since, in India, he had liver complaints, for which he used quantities of mercury, and dispersed an abscess which it was expected would break. The mercurial course appeared to him to have altogether unsettled the tone and functions of the alimentary canal; which from that time had always been in a state of excessive irritability, and generally in excessive action also. I remarked, that much would depend on his carefully avoiding those things, that by experience he knew would disagree with him; to which he replied, it was difficult to resist temptation, for that it was only a day or two since he had been made very ill by eating toasted cheese in ale, of which he was excessively fond. He said he had tried bitters and astringents without benefit; and was anxious to know my opinion whether there was ulceration of the mucous coat of the bowels, or any other organic disease.

He observed, that eighteen months since he had consulted a surgeon of high celebrity, who had examined the rectum by the finger, told him there was an ulcer in the bowel, and even made a drawing for him upon paper, to show him its exact figure, directing a lotion to be injected over the part. Mr. WHITE, of Bath, had since examined him, and assured him he did not believe an ulcer existed then, whatever there might have been before; and that, as to stricture, he passed a bougie eleven or twelve inches without finding any.

He complained that he was almost constantly teased to pass motions, especially in the morning; but that by washing out the rectum with warm milk and water, be generally removed the uneasiness; and might pass a quiet day, if at home. But that if, from being absent at a friend's house, he was prevented using his apparatus, the urgency of the tenesmus increased, exposing him to much distress and misery. The discharges were rarely bilious, generally a frothy mucus; never bloody, except now and then to a trifling degree, from severe straining. On examination, I found the mucous membrane of the gut relaxed, and thrown into folds; with a tenderness just perceptible, towards the prostate gland.

The opinion I gave was, that I had known, in more than one instance, all his present symptoms arise from diarrhœa, where there was no proof of ulceration, nor in fact of any other organic disease, for the patients recovered perfectly; and that I, therefore, thought he had no good ground for his suspicions, his complaints being rather connected with function than structure. They were, however, no less important on that account, for without making large concessions to them, particularly in what related to diet and management, and that for several years to come, I was very sure, from my knowledge of these complaints, he would never get rid of them; although, on the other hand, if he chose to live by rule, and avail himself of the assistance of medicine, when it might be capable of benefiting him, I was equally certain that by degrees his complaints might be removed, and his health perfectly restored.

Case 25.

Scirrhous Uterus, simulating deranged Bowels.

Mrs. Chidlow, an elderly woman, consulted me regarding a complaint to which she was very subject. Her disorder was a bearing down, and great pain in her back and loins, restlessness, want of appetite, great irritability of stomach, and prostration of strength. The pulse was quick, and small. Pressure on the abdomen gave no pain. Occasionally an irritable diarrhœa came on; at other times she was constipated with urgent desire to evacuate. Puzzled as to the immediate seat of disease, I examined the rectum, and found the uterus projecting and enlarged, with its fundus of a scirrous stony hardness.

Some leeches were applied to her back; and

the alimentary canal acted upon by occasional laxatives and clysters. By attention to these means she was made comfortable in her attacks, and allowed a longer respite from invasion.

Case 26.

Irritable Rectum from diseased Womb.

A poor woman, aged 42, requested assistance from the St. George's Infirmary, Nov. 7. 1820. She dated the commencement of her illness from her last lying in, five years before. She was, on that occasion, attended by a person sent from a public charity, who neglected her both in and after her labour. Exhausted with the fatigue of her pains, she was left previous to the separation of the placenta, and falling asleep for half an hour, awoke, cold, and shivering, as if in the most violent ague. She was, however, laid under warm blankets, became warm, and sweated profusely. For several days she was unable to move in bed, from the tender and extremely painful state of the abdomen. She had also feverish heat, thirst, and several nights dilirium. Although, after the first week, (being totally unattended,) she endeavoured to leave her bed, she felt so extremely sore about the stomach as to be scarcely able to bear the bed-clothes; and in the sixth week, in the attempt to go to church, she fainted away, and was unable to get out of the house.

As to her medical treatment, she said she had only once been ordered medicine, and that was some castor-oil; her medical attendant paid her only three visits in the first fortnight, and then left her altogether. Notwithstanding these difficulties, she nursed and suckled her infant.

From this period she was subject, particularly in cold weather, to sudden and severe rigors, with cold sweats, followed by a feverish paroxysm, head-ach, heat of skin, and thirst. The violent shaking usually ceased on getting into a warm bed; but she generally remained cold after this for an hour or two. These attacks would return sometimes twice in the day, and sometimes only once in a fortnight; they always began with a sense of cold in the region of the womb; thence appearing to spread over the whole body.

About a year after her confinement, in addition to the above complaints, she took cold, and soon after this felt a sensation as of strings passing up from the navel to the chest, drawn tight by the motions of respiration. Within the last six months she had felt as if these strings were drawn tighter than before; several of them produced much distress, drawing or pulling from the navel down to the hip and upwards to the chest, whenever she coughed. At these points she sometimes felt extremely sore and tender, particularly when so unfortunate as to have cough or cold-

In May, 1820, she experienced symptoms of approaching disease in the womb, severe pains at the loins, uneasiness in the thighs and hips, sense of swelling, a constant bearing down in the region of the womb, and deficient menstrnation. About this period, also, she first observed that the passage of the fæces along the bowel for some distance above the anus gave pain. She was then in the country for her health, but some weeks after, returning to town, a diarrhœa came on, which, although it prevented the pain incident to confined stools, incurred a degree of tenesmus nearly as bad. The motions were thin, mucus, and tinged with blood, neither offensive, nor in the least degree bilious. Upon her recovery from the looseness, the uneasy and painful state of the bowel seemed to be somewhat relieved.

In November she observed that she still felt the uneasy sensations in her inside, as if strings or cords, two or three of which felt as if attached to the left groin, extending from the navel. She uniformly found them most troublesome when loose and undressed in bed, the pressure of the stays appearing to restrain and support the abdomen, and prevent them from pulling.

By examination, the womb was found considerably enlarged, and very irritable. The rectum in its structure was sound; but the mucus membrane, for as far as the finger would reach, was extremely tender and irritable, especially on its anterior part.

With regard to treatment, the peculiar febrile paroxysms to which she was subject were found to be most effectually relieved by full doses of the compound powder of ipecacuan.; a plan which, under some modification, appeared to be most suitable to the alleviation of her uterine complaints. The irritable state of the rectum, when particularly troublesome, was very much relieved and composed, by the occasional use of an anodyne injection, consisting of half a pint of warm barley-water, or thin gruel, with thirty drops of tincture of opium. Sometimes, although rarely, I had directed a larger quantity of laudanum; but it was apt to leave confinement, followed by subsequent increase of irritation.

Case 27.

Irritable Rectum from diseased Womb.

Nov. 1. 1820. I was requested to see a female aged 55, who for some years had been distressed with piles, which occasionally bled freely; they were now rarely troublesome. For the last three months she had been afflicted with severe pains in the loins, which, in their progress, settled down into the left hip and thigh, where they became intense, and constant. These complaints had been followed by tenderness and soreness about the anus; with occasional pain and frequency in making water. The most severe pain occurred in passing a motion, particularly if the fæces were at all hard. This pain was not in the anus, but in the bowel, some distance above.

She observed, she had been attended by a medical gentleman, who, upon hearing of a difficulty and pain in her evacuations, had at once decided there was a stricture, to remove which he had passed up a large-sized bougie, a procedure which threw her into such an agony of pain, that she was sure she had never been so well since.

On examination, several small flaccid tumors were found at the verge of the anus, the mucous membrane within the bowel, and the general structure of the intestine were apparently sound, but so irritable, that the lightest motion of the finger over any part of the surface, threw the whole frame into tremor and agitation. This irritable condition of the bowel was clearly consequent to disease in its neighbourhood, for there was a large tuberculated tumor that might be felt through the coats of the intestine, evidently a disease of the womb; not only accounting for the affection of the bowel, but that of the bladder also. The vagina was next examined; its cavity was shortened, its parietes thickened, giving the impression of an irregular induration; besides which, it was partially closed, apparently in consequence of inflammation with effusion of lymph and the subsequent formation of transverse and oblique bands within its canal. She expressed an anxious hope that I should not think it necessary to use instruments; upon which point I at once set her mind at rest, by stating my conviction that in her case instruments would not only prove useless but injurious.

Nov. 8. She said, that about two years since she was much distressed by a discharge from the vagina, at first pale, but afterward frequently tinged with blood, for many weeks attended with exteme irritation and pain in making water, and constant sense of great heat in the parts. This complaint was productive of feverish heat, and so much languor, that sometimes she was ready to faint with exhaustion: it continued nearly six months, and appears to have been the period when the effusion of coagulable lymph took place in the vagina.

Jan. 22, 1821. The irritable state of the rectum and of the uterine tumor, were constant sources of apprehension and dread. She experienced more torment than ever in passing her motions, notwithstanding the bowels were regulated with the greatest care. There was no change observed by examination of the intestine, although in other points the disease was extending itself, there being now complete retraction and numbness of the left thigh. Opiates, ætherial, and other antispasmodic medicines, forming the basis of her treatment, produced considerable relief to the uneasy state of the bowel.

Case 28.

Ulcerated Opening into the intestines, from an Abscess.

A. G. aged twenty-two, left her place in January, 1814, with severe pain in the left side of the abdomen, and went into St. George's Hospital, where, by frequent bleedings and much care, she was in four months relieved, and discharged. She attended a family to Lisbon, but frequently felt the old pain in the old spot, with a sense of swelling inwardly, and acute or throbbing pain.

June, 1816, she came into the St. George's Infirmary for venereal eruptions, of which, by mercurial frictions she was cured. A considerable excitement, on this occasion, produced neither pain nor change in the internal tumour, which seemed to vary in size, but was generally, to her feelings, equal to a large orange. Soon after she left the house the swelling enlarged, with a burning heat and throbbing, and a flush of inflammation on the corresponding part of the external integuments.

In October, she again came into the Infirmary; supposed pregnant; but tenderness, local pain, and being perfectly regular, made it improbable. The internal heat and throbbing increaesd daily, with extreme tenderness, and much pain in taking a deep inspiration.

She was blistered and leached repeatedly, to no purpose. The blisters having excited execssive irritation, formentations were applied, and continued till December 30., when, after increased suffering, she became uncommonly easy, felt sick at the stomach, and presently vomited a quantity of blood and pus. The sickness repeatedly returned, and in the course of the day she threw up nearly a quart of the same kind of matter; and also passed several stools, similar to what had been rejected by vomiting.

The occasional returns of vomiting, or purging, or both, brought away frequent and large quantities of offensive purulent matter, streaked with blood; and thus continued till July, 1817, when they finally left her, under the use of various tonic medicines, by which she was restored to perfect health. In the following year she became pregnant, and was safely delivered of a large and healthy child.

CASE 29.

*Ulceration of the Colon.**

Sir S. M., in the year 1780, fell from the deck of his ship, and struck his side violently against the edge of a boat lying alongside. By this accident he was confined, and it was many months before he was well enough to stand upright. This difficulty by degrees wore off, but he remained ever after liable to occasional pains in the part. Subsequent to this accident he was for many years before his death subject to gout, weak bowels, depraved appetite, and a winter cough.

In February, 1795, he was much exposed to the cold of a very severe winter, and to use his own words, "he felt his bowels chilled;" from this

* Extracted from the MS history in Mr. HEAVISIDE's museum, where the disease is preserved.

time he was never well. It was thought to be suppressed gout, and he went to Bath for ten weeks, to no purpose. Almost every night he had now great pain in the bowels. From these attacks he was generally relieved upon passing two or three motions, more or less purulent.

Thus he went on, having alternately, as he described them, two kinds of pain; one a grinding, gnawing, and oppressive pain; the other, (which always preceded a motion,) of the common griping kind. Latterly, both these kinds of pain came on in an aggravated degree every second or third day; then, by giving a purge, a great quantity of offensive purulent fæces were brought away, relieving him for a few days till his pains returned. His sufferings increased; he continued to languish only till the following October, when he died.

On examination, the viscera of the abdomen in general were found tolerably healthy; the principal disease being confined to the lower end of the ileum, cœcum, and especially the colon, in that part of its arch directly under the part where the bruise had been received fifteen years before. The whole length of the colon had suffered inflammation, and this had connected itself with ulceration through the whole extent of the mucous membrane of the bowel, the coats of which were three or four times their natural thickness, the diameter of the canal being diminished in the same proportion.

Case 30.

Ulcer in the Rectum.

A gentleman, aged thirty-two, visited London for advice. He complained of constant pain, and soreness about the anus, with frequent returns of tenesmus and bearing down. On examination, I found two small hæmorrhoidal swellings at the side of the arms. At one part the surface was ulcerated, and the ulcer, partly external, extended itself for some distance within the sphincter. His physician directed such medicines as were best suited to improve tone, and restore strength in a weak and irritable constitution. During several weeks various local applications were tried without benefit. Dry lint was then used alone; the surface improved, but did not heal. The lint was now dipped in a solution of five grains of the argentum nitratum, in an ounce of water. This produced a smarting pain, but its good effect was soon made manifest, for in three days new skin began to form; in a fortnight most of the external ulcer was cicatrized; and in a month more, that part of it within the sphincter was also healed. This might have been presumed, by the relief experienced from irritation and tenesmus, but it was proved by examining the parts when protruded.

Case 31.

Hæmorrhage from the Bowels; from Ulceration.

A thin healthy young woman, hanging cloaths from a second-floor window, over-reached herself, the line broke, dragged her out, and she fell on her side, with a twist of the back, upon the stones of a stable yard. I visited her the same day (Oct. 18, 1820), and directed a large blister to her side, and an opening mixture. She said that in the fall, the end of the strong busk of her stays, pushed violently in just above the bladder towards the back-bone, and at this point, which appeared to be about the middle of the arch of the colon, pressure was painful. For the first week I persuaded her to keep herself abstinent, relaxed, and quiet; and had a second blister applied.

Nov. 6. For a day or two after the accident the pain on pressure, where the back had been bruised, was distressing, but this relieved by the blister she felt no more of it till Nov. 2, (the 16th day;) on this day she had been washing, and supposed she might possibly have strained herself, when towards evening she felt violent shooting, and prickling pains, her back and loins being worse than usual, with tenesmus, which, only a quarter of an hour after the pain began in the bowels, induced her to think she could pass a motion, but she only parted with more than half a pint of dark, coagulated blood, without other matter.

ULCERATION. 115

Easier for an hour, she then felt the same pains return with a sensation of prickling and pinching, neither higher nor lower than the original spot, but extended occasionally a hand-breadth laterally. The second attack was about ten at night, and from this she was somewhat relieved by voiding half a tea-cup full of blood. The pains were so distressing, as to render her watchful and feverish: afraid to cough, sneeze, and even to breathe, on account of the pain.

The following morning, she took an opening powder, and this, in a quarter of an hour, relieved her greatly, upon her passing about half a pint of red, and fluid blood; she remained easier all the day, but on the return of night got little sleep, and that very disturbed.

Nov. 4. She made known what had happened, and I directed the infusion of roses to be taken frequently; this in two days set her so perfectly to rights, that she had no return of bleeding or pain, nor felt the least uneasiness on moderate pressure.

In this instance it appears to me, from the circumstances of the case, the bleeding came from the intestines, and that the part injured was the transverse arch of the colon; it also appears to me that the most probable cause of the bleeding, was the separation or sloughing of the bruised internal surface of the bowel, which in casting off had opened vessels of sufficient consequence to furnish the hæmorrhage that followed. The manner and course of the symptoms leave little room for doubt upon this point; and considering it as established, it is worthy of remark, that the part so soon assumed healthy action; as the patient only four days after the bleeding experienced no local inconvenience in any one respect, nor the least uneasiness in any part of her bowels, even under pressure.

Case 32.

Ulceration with Tumour in the Rectum.

J. Earle, aged sixty-three, after having been several years subject to diarrhœa, for many months to constant pain in the loins, and still more lately to a severe pain in the rectum, opposite the middle of the sacrum, was admitted, under the physician's care, into the St. George's Infirmary, where he became exceedingly emaciated, and at length died, exhausted by constant pain and irritation. The stools latterly were as frequent as every hour, although he took scarcely any support; the motions were generally fluid, but rarely fæcal. About three months before his death, the rectum had been examined, but nothing particular was ascertained.

Dr. JAMES, who had paid the most humane attention to the poor man through his illness, considering his complaints had not been perfectly understood, requested the body might be opened. The examination was made January 29. 1819. On opening the abdomen, a circumscribed tumour, the size of an hen's egg, was felt within the rectum;

the bowel was therefore removed and opened. The lower end of the intestine for the space of five inches above the sphincter was healthy, and consequently the disease could not have been felt in examining per anum.

The disease itself consisted of two flattened tumours, apparently a deposit in the cellular texture, between the inner membrane and the muscular coat, which, by pressing the two sides of the gut together, might have partially impeded the passage of contents, although the bowels were found empty.

The irritation from this disease must have been great, for one of the inner surfaces had ulcerated into a deep cavity, the mucous membrane round the margin of the ulcer being thickened and pulpy and its texture rendered indeterminate by small specks of blood effused into its substance. The projecting edges of the ulcer lay beyond the basis of the tumour within the intestine. On dividing through the substance of the tumour it was in some parts firm and compact, as if small tubercular deposits of fatty, white-coloured matter had taken place into the cellular membrane. The muscular coat was perfectly healthy.

CHAPTER III.

ON THE GROWTH OF TUMOURS WITHIN THE BOWEL.

SECT. 1.

On the Causes of the Disease.

110. THE formation of tumours within the rectum is not a frequent consequence of disease. When it does occur, it is sometimes beyond the reach of surgery to remove, or even relieve. Occasionally, it is otherwise. I have seen several instances of disease of this kind, of which I have not preserved accurate notes. In one of these, had the patient felt sufficient confidence in the means proposed for his relief, an operation might have been performed with success. The late Mr. HEY of Leeds has published a case of this kind. These remarks will show the importance of considering and discriminating this disease in practice.

111. The determining the particular cause that may have produced any complaint of this description will generally be difficult. In a few instances it would appear to be referable to some

mechanical irritation, disturbing the healthy actions of the part. In one case it followed the operation for fistula in ano; but most commonly it would appear that a latent disposition, either in the part or the constitution, is merely called into action by some local irritation.

112. M. DESAULT considered the formation of tumours and obstructions in the rectum as frequently caused by venereal complaints imperfectly cured. He styles them scirrhous affections; but, I presume, it may be taken for granted that he renders the term rather comprehensive than correct, since he relates, under this title, two cases, both of which were cured by compression only.

That disease of this, or indeed of any other kind, may sometimes occur in those who have formerly had venereal complaints, is so clear, that this circumstance seems to afford a very inconclusive argument in favour of any necessary connection; and even should mercury, under suspicion of venereal taint, have been employed, and that with success, it still appears to me that, considering how frequently the mercurial stimulus has excited absorption in other diseases, there will be much stronger ground for determining that the complaint was not scirrhous, than for asserting that it was venereal.

Sect. 2.

On the Symptoms and Appearances.

113. The early progress of tumours in the rectum will rarely excite much attention; particularly as the functions and feelings incident to the bowels are occasionally subject to considerable variation, even in perfect health.

The first circumstance, perhaps, that may draw the attention, may be a sense of local uneasiness, or pain: but this symptom, as far as I have seen, having been always connected, either with confinement or relaxation of bowels, the inconvenience has been naturally attributed to the only obvious cause; and the means adopted under this impression succeed at first relieving, if not removing the complaint.

114. These remarks, however, apply only to tumours formed between the coats of the intestine, and even in these there will be exceptions, where the disease assumes the appearances and follows the usual course of scrophula in other parts.

When a tumour is projected from the inner membrane of the gut, attached by a narrow neck, I have known it reach the size of a large chesnut, without any symptom, except trifling pain in passing a confined motion.

M. Delpech mentions an instance in which several tumours of this kind, in the rectum, excited tenesmus and frequent griping pains in the bowels.

Upon one of these occasions the violent contractions of the intestine ruptured the neck of one of the tumours, which, voided by the anus, led to examination of the parts, and the consequent detection of the disease.

115. In the progress of the complaint, symptoms became more distinct; and, provided the disease is situated between the coats of the intestine, and has, consequently, an intimate connection with the surrounding structure, there will, in some cases, be constant uneasiness, or sense of weight, or occasional paroxysms of pain about the sacrum. When, on the other hand, the patient is only incommoded by occasional obstruction to the passage of the fæces, the tumour will generally be found so attached as to admit of removal by an operation.

116. In the advanced stages, where the disease has been extensively diffused through the cellular membrane, I have seen frequent and sometimes excessive hæmorrhage from the external surface of a soft tubercular mass, the blood not having been effused from an ulcerated part, but poured out by the exhalent arteries dispersed upon the surface of the disease. Under these circumstances the blood accumulates in the rectum, till, exciting a painful spasm, it is expelled, and the patient relieved.

117. I have seen one specimen of tumour formed between the coats of the intestine ileum, projecting inward so as to occupy the whole natural space of the bowel; and consequently as it must have absolutely obstructed the passage of fæces,

it most probably from this cause terminated fatally. The size of the tumour is that of a small apple, the base is broad; it is covered by the inner membrane of the bowel, and where it is divided, exhibits a very compact scirrhous structure. The preparation is in Dr. HOOPER's select and valuable collection of diseases.

118. I once examined a person having a tumour in the rectum, attached by a narrow neck, about three inches above the sphincter. It gave no pain under examination, was moderately firm, but appeared to be softest towards the surface, from which there had been repeated bleeding. In this case, although the disease was hæmorrhagic, and had excited tenesmus, it was painless, and might have been safely removed.

119. One of the most distressing symptoms produced by tumours in this situation, is the consequence of irritation from sympathy of parts. Sooner or later an irksome diarrhœa takes place, from the increased quantity of fluids poured into the bowels; a complaint that, while it harasses the patient, diminishes his strength, and eventnally renders the stomach irritable, and incapable of its proper functions.

120. The structure of many of these tumours exhibits exactly the appearances that are observed in scirrhous affections in other parts of the body. The scirrhous tumour seated in the coats of the intestine, and projecting into the cavity, I have seen, but believe it to be extremely rare. The soft tumour I have found, in connection with similar disease, either in the bladder, in the male, or the uterus in the female.

Sect 3.

On the Treatment.

121. The first object in this as in all other diseases, must be to obtain a clear and correct knowledge of all its circumstances. The practitioner, therefore, when from symptoms he is led to suspect the seat of the complaint, must point out the necessity for making more particular enquiry, in the way of examination, as the only means by which a clear idea can be obtained regarding the figure, firmness, irritability, or sensibility of the disease. By these means alone can the information be acquired which is necessary, for the deciding whether the affection is, or is not, of such nature as to admit or require being relieved or removed by an operation.

122. Where a tumour is found to be small in size, of moderately firm texture, and not painful under gentle pressure, benefit may probably be derived from the occasional introduction of an instrument capable of making a degree of pressure. In some circumstances, this purpose may be answered by the elastic gum bougie, in others the mode recommended by M. Desault may be preferred, a bougie of lint supported by a concealed probe, being at intervals allowed to remain for a time in contact with the tumour. Whatever instrument is used, the degree of pres-

sure, and the frequency of its repetition, must be regulated with care, according to the patient's feelings, and the tendency manifested by the disease.

123. The disease may on examination be found to possess the firmness of scirrhus, or it may, on the contrary, have the soft consistence of fungus hæmatodes. In either state the use of bougies will be more likely to aggravate than to arrest the progress of the complaint. In both these forms of disease, the only principle to be kept in view, is that of attending diligently to the daily progress of symptoms, endeavouring to relieve them as they occur, either by the judicious exhibition of opiates or some other of the means mentioned as appropriate for the treatment of stricture. (61.)

124. The soft pulpy tumour generally becomes, sooner or later, subject to hæmorrhage; this is consequently a circumstance that may at any time require attention. The object, however, is merely that of restraining a flux of blood, without expecting the removal of the cause by any thing that can be proposed in the way of treatment. The present loss of blood may be generally arrested, by directing a strong astringent injection to be thrown up. This may, according to circumstances, be an infusion of roses, decoction of oak-bark, of the rind of the pomegranate, or strong infusion of galls; any of these may be rendered more powerful by the addition of a concentrated aluminous solution.

125. When, from the irritation of the disease, nausea, vomiting, or diarrhœa supervene, medicines must be directed to quiet these complaints.

The most useful remedies for this purpose are opiates and aromatics.

126. The appearance of purulent matter in the stools certainly argues the existence of ulceration; but whether the ulcerated surface is exposed towards the cavity of the gut, or otherwise, can only be known by an examination per anum, the most satisfactory of all methods of enquiry, where the seat of the affection is within reach of the finger.

127. Suppose the disease is known to have ulcerated, I am not acquainted with any plan of treatment that has much chance of success; as, however, it is our duty to attempt something, I should recommend those means that might operate through the medium of the constitution, either with a view to improve strength and moderate excessive action (101.), or diminish excessive irritability, according to circumstances.

128. Should the tumour be such as to admit of removal by an operation (114.), the ligature may be recommended. Preparatory to its application, it will, however, be right to empty the bowels. As to the particular mode of applying the ligature, no specific direction can be given. When the tumour is large, or its attachment high up, advantage may be gained in the freedom of operating by dilating the sphincter, by the previous introduction of sponge tent. A few weeks since, I removed by ligature a tumour the size of a large cherry, growing by a narrow neck from the internal surface of the rectum, in a child nine years old; situated so low down

as to admit of its being brought out by straining. In consistence, it was firm, but not scirrhous; neither was the operation painful.

129. In the application of the ligature, the manner which I think best, from having found it most convenient in the extirpation of an exceedingly enlarged tonsil, is that recommended by Ambrose Pare. It is a simple ligature of sufficient strength, with a running noose at one end; this adjusted round the basis of the tumour, the loop is tightened by an instrument with a small string that runs freely over the line, pushing the knot before it, and consequently diminishing the noose, or tightening the ligature to the degree required. In some circumstances, perhaps, the ligature may be better applied by a canula.

130. Any tendency to inflammation previous to the dropping off of the ligature, may be checked or regulated by occasional warm emollient injections, assisted by fomentations externally.

M. Desault mentions his having removed by ligature a tumour of this kind the size of a hen's egg; its attachment was near six inches above the anus; the ligature came away on the eighth day, and the patient did well.

131. Where the tumour is within view, M. Desault recommends the ligature to be first secured, and the tumour then cut off, to avoid the offence from its mortifying, and the injury that might arise from excoriation of surrounding parts. These reasons, however, are not of sufficient weight to counterbalance what has al-

ways appeared to me objectionable in the practice. It is clear that any living part falling into a state of decay, must be offensive; but it is to me equally clear, and that from long observation, that when a part is thus destroyed, the perfect mortification of the dead part assists in completing that process of vitality by which the ligature is separated; and as the application of a ligature now and then excites much constitutional irritation, so is it an object that may regard even the safety of the patient, to attend to every circumstance that may assist in expediting that ulceration by which the ligature is to be eventually thrown off.

CHAPTER IV.

ON PROLAPSUS ANI.

Sect. I.

On the Causes of the Disease.

132. The verge of the anus, surrounded by a strong band of muscular fibres, and supported in its place by other muscular expansions, is occasionally subject to relaxation; and any circumstance that favors this relaxation may become a cause of prolapsus ani.

133. Disordered states of the bowels are among the most frequent causes of this complaint. Diarrhœa, by weakening the constitution, and particularly the intestinal canal, is sometimes the means of inducing prolapsus ani, although it is more commonly brought on by attacks of cholera morbus, or dysentery. The irritation from worms, or the rough operation of drastic purgatives, will not unfrequently produce it. I have seen several instances of this in children, and was very lately consulted by a young lady, who, when a child, had been subject to worms,

for which her mamma was persuaded to give her a patent worm medicine; it operated so violently as to produce a prolapsus ani, to which she has ever since remained subject.

134. One of the most formidable instances I ever witnessed of this infirmity was in 1815, in a poor man, forty-one years of age, in whom it was brought on, together with the more common symptoms of colica pictonum by working many years at his business as a house painter.

135. Habitual confinement of bowels, and the occasional straining incident to such state, are frequent causes of prolapsus. The pressure of the gravid uterus, by impeding the functions of the bowels, or any other circumstances that either prevent their regular action, or induce violent efforts, will bring on this complaint. The severe pains of labour favour its production, and especially the straining and tenesmus occasioned by an irritable bladder, whether this is dependent on stricture in the urethra, stone, diseased prostate gland, or any other cause.

SECT. 2.

On the Symptoms and Appearances.

136. THE order of the symptoms is subject to much variation. In some the disease appears suddenly, in others its approach is almost imperceptible. In young children, who either from having been too long kept at the breast, or from bad diet, possess a weakened and relaxed fibre, it

commonly appears to arise from mere debility in the sphincter, which giving way, allows the bowel to be suddenly protruded, sometimes to a considerable extent. In grown persons, however, I have scarcely ever seen it take place in this manner; it is most commonly produced by slow degrees. In the efforts to relieve the bowels a fulness is usually first observed about the anus; soon after this, a thin fold of the inner membrane of the gut, generally very vascular, may be perceived to protrude; and this becomes more manifest, till at length a tumour of considerable bulk is formed. This tumour, at first only a production of the inner membrane, subsequently consists of a portion of the entire bowel, protruded completely beyond the verge of the anus. The degree of protrusion may be such as to show that, although the bowel is connected by its peritoneal covering, as well as by its blood-vessels, to the spine, these parts are occasionally capable of great relaxation, where the complaint is gradually formed. I have, in various instances, seen in young children the prolapsed part of the bowel produce a tumour four or five inches in length; and in the adult subject, especially in aged persons, have found the volume of the protrusion exceed the size of a large orange. A late writer speaks of an extent including several feet of intestine being thus circumstanced;* but this must be regarded as, at least, a very unusual occurrence.

* M. Delpech.

137. In the examination necessarily connected with the reduction of these tumours, it has frequently appeared to me that the protrusion, although favoured by a relaxed sphincter, has been partly the consequence of relaxation in the coats of the bowel itself. I was very lately able to confirm the accuracy of this opinion by examining the body of a man who died of apoplexy, and who, for years, had been subject to a prolapsus of the rectum. On laying open the abdomen, the intestines in general where not deficient in tone; the rectum and anus were removed. For near six inches the bowel was enlarged. The superior part of the intestine, contracted and firm, did not exceed the diameter of half an inch; the inferior, relaxed, flaccid, and unresising, was nearly three inches in diameter. As the whole of the intestine was empty, the comparative state of its different parts was more readily determined; and it was evident that, while the upper part had retained its healthy tone, the lower portion had long lost its power of action, or resistance, and was subject to every impression, either from contents or surrounding parts. The muscular fibres of the longitudinal bands, perfect upon the contracted were dispersed and lost on reaching the dilated portion of the intestine. The volume of the relaxed part of the bowel about equalled the quantity I had on one occasion found protruded, when requested to visit him, about five months before his death.

138. In its natural state, the internal surface of the rectum is soft, tender, and moist; but I have

more than once, in persons who were in years, found the protruded part of the gut, by long exposure, very much thickened, of more firm texture, and dry; appearing in fact like a part covered with strong integuments.

139. In one instance, a small extent of the lower extremity of the bowel remaining permanently protruded, afforded me the opportunity of watching the progressive change by which the fine mucous membrane became converted, as it were, into a part of the external integument.* Neither is this power of accommodation, this facility in changing its character according to circumstances, a gift bestowed only upon the inner surface of the rectum; a case is recorded in which a part of the colon was wounded, and protruded for many years in a state of inversion, upon the left side of the belly; the protruded gut would bear washing with the greatest freedom, with ice and snow water, in the coldest weather; and the effect of exposure to the cold air, was only to render it contracted, hardened, and of a paler colour.† Where this change has taken place to any considerable extent, I have not found reduction always practicable. M. LIEUTAUD seems to have met with this state of parts, which he terms scirrhous: he says, "La partie du rectum deplacee devient quelquefois squirrheuse; et l'on a alors beaucoup de peine a la faire rentrer."‡

---

* Case 39.   † Phil. Trans. vol. xxxi.
‡ Précis de la Medecine, tom. iii.

140. Where the sphincter has not entirely lost its power of action, the constriction may produce either a partial or total arrest of circulation in the prolapsed parts, inducing mortification. The risk of this event forms one of the strongest reasons in favour of immediate reduction, in most tumours of this description.

141. Prolapsus, although it may not induce total arrest of circulation, is generally productive of difficulty in the return of the venous blood; on some occasions the over-distended veins may be seen exposed, and may be observed to be unable to relieve themselves, and in this embarrassment, the powers of the constitution, ever active in removing evil where prevention fails, have been watched; while, without the least disturbance to the system, the varicose vessels have sloughed away, and the parts have readily healed up as if nothing of the least importance had occurred.*

142. It now and then happens that complaints similar to the above in external appearance, but of a more complicated nature, fall under observation; and unless the practitioner is previously aware of the exact relation that the one case bears to the other, he will not discern accurately between them, and will certainly not adopt the curative means most likely to succeed.

143. The intestinal canal, a continued tube possessing peculiar powers, may be expected to be

---

* Case 39.

subject to peculiar affections. It is susceptible of partial and transitory contraction, is highly elastic, and generally contains air more or less extensively diffused through its cavity. Owing to these and other circumstances, it is occasionally exposed to an accident that cannot occur to any other part of the body. It is liable to have one part of its tube thrust forward, as it were, into that which is immediately before it, in the course of the canal, forming an intus-susception.

144. This accident in young children, while the parts still retain much of their original tone, is sometimes extremely dangerous, and when it produces symptoms, it generally terminates fatally; but in grown persons I have frequently ascertained its existence in examination after death without any reason for thinking it had produced inconvenience, much less danger, owing, as I believe, to the gradual diminution of tone, which very commonly renders the bowels, in advanced age, indisposed even to the requisite degree of action in the regular propulsion of their contents.

145. The manner in which the small intestine ileum terminates, by insertion into the comparatively large head of the colon, will in some degree explain why the former part is now and then found included within the latter: where the circumstances producing this kind of derangement continue to operate, the displacement may go on increasing to an astonishing extent. I have, in several instances, found a considerable portion of the colon, together with the cœcum, and part of

the ileum, included within the lower end of the colon and rectum.*

146. Should this peculiar state of parts occur, in conjunction with relaxation of the sphincter, there is nothing to prevent the inverted part of the bowel within the rectum protruding outwardly. This protrusion has taken place, and it is very important to know also that it has most frequently been mistaken for a common prolapsus ani. Provided, however, the practitioner has previously formed a clear idea of the two cases, and the exact relation the one bears to the other, there will be no difficulty in at once distinguishing them.

147. In the prolapsus ani, the lower end of the bowel, or that directly above the sphincter muscle, will be first protruded; it will be inverted, and confine within it a corresponding extent of the uninverted gut next above it. Now, if in examination, a probe be introduced between the circle of the relaxed sphincter and that of the prolapsed bowel, it will of course be prevented passing inward by the position of the parts, the rectum being folded down immediately within the anus.

In intus-susception, on the other hand, the rectum is no further concerned than in having permitted the superior part of the bowel to pass into its cavity, and consequently if the portion of intestine that may have protruded through the anus be examined, a probe may, with the utmost ease, be passed freely up between the sphincter

* Case 41.

and internal surface of the rectum, and the apposed surface of the inverted colon, and may also, without the least difficulty, be passed freely round the whole circle of the sphincter, between it and the prolapsed intestine.

This distinction is of much practical importance; the want of it may involve the character of the practitioner, and will infinitely diminish the chance of recovery to the patient.

148. Where intus-susception has taken place to such an extent, as to have brought down the small into the large intestine, and particularly where the bowel so circumstanced is protruded beyond the anus, it constitutes a case of the most serious and critical description, compared with a mere prolapsus of the anus. The difficulty and uncertainty of the event in any attempt at the replacement in the first case is infinitely great, while in the second, there is commonly little or no difficulty at all.

Sect. 3.

On the Treatment.

149. The particular nature of the cause will determine the treatment required for the removal of prolapsus ani. Where it occurs in infancy or early youth, as the result of extreme laxity of fibre from too long suckling, it is scarcely necessary to observe, that till the child is weaned, no plan of cure is worth the trial. Should a similar state of

constitution have been favoured by a poor and unwholesome diet, this point also must of course be regarded in the treatment. The state of the habit must be corrected by the use of tonicks, as bark, steel, and the cold bath, aided by an appropriate regimen. Under this plan, with constant attention to preserve regularity in the action of the bowels, the protrusion will often become less considerable, less frequent, and will eventually cease to return at all.

150. Prolapsus now and then occurs under the operation of drastic purgatives, where there is no natural disposition to the complaint, for which the required treatment will be some attention to rest, and more to the avoiding the re-application of the cause, by any immoderate irritation of the bowels.

151. Where prolapsus in the adult has been brought on by diarrhœa, dysentery, or colica pictonum, attention may be required for the local complaint, but no material step can be taken toward its cure, till the disorder of the bowels is removed, or the constitutional state corrected.

152. Prolapsus, connected with labour pains, is generally of temporary duration; the cause upon which it depends being transitory, the parts generally soon recover themselves.

153. In reducing a prolapsus ani, the application of gentle pressure; the fingers being previously moistened with oil, is usually all that is necessary; it frequently happens that if the patient reclines on a sofa or bed for half an hour, this alone will enable the parts to recover themselves.

or should the prolapsus not return spontaneously it may then be reduced in the manner above-mentioned.

154. When, from neglect or other cause, the quantity of the protrusion has become considerable, its reduction may not prove so easy. The object in operating must then be to return that part first, which was last pushed down, to effect which, one of the fingers may be gently insinuated into the cavity of the protruded bowel, and may be made very useful in facilitating the reduction of the prolapsus; these endeavours of the operator being assisted by maintaining a steady and equal pressure upon the other parts of the tumour.

155. Should inflammation and constriction have taken place, active measures will be necessary for the prevention of serious mischief to the bowel, which, unless relieved, may fall into a state of gangrene. Immersion in the warm bath may here prove useful, it will favour relaxation, and sometimes render reduction practicable. If this should not succeed, leeches or cupping-glasses may be applied in the immediate vicinity of the parts and the warm bath or fomentations be then repeated. By these means I believe almost every prolapsus of the rectum may be safely returned, at least I have only once seen them fail, and then it was owing to the long neglect of the patient, from which the protruded bowel had become excessively thickened and indurated.

156. Should any enlarged veins be found upon the inverted part of the prolapsus, the use of mild fomentations will be the best treatment; whether

they remain in apparent health, or perhaps manifest a disposition to slough out in the manner already adverted to. (141.)

157. Tonic and astringent applications, as fomentations or injections, have been directed by various authors for the relief of prolapsus; but having often tried these means without material advantage, I now very rarely recommend them. Instruments for keeping up the parts are almost entirely useless.

158. I shall now point out what appears to me to be the best mode of curing this disease, by an operation.

In the year 1802, I assisted Mr. HEAVISIDE in removing some hæmorrhoidal tumours. The patient was a gentleman who had come up from the country for advice. Three ligatures were applied, and the consequent inflammation was considerable. The benefit derived from the operation exceeded expectation, for upon his recovery he mentioned that he had for some time been subject not only to the swellings now removed, but also to a protrusion of the bowel whenever he went to stool, but that since the operation, this symptom had entirely disappeared.

159. This circumstance struck my attention, and on seeing the observations subsequently published by the late Mr. HEY, of Leeds, the conclusion I had formed, as to the above case, was confirmed. Mr. HEY was consulted for a prolapsus ani; and, finding the sphincter surrounded by a pendulous flap and other protuberances, he determined to remove them, " in

the hope that the inflammation caused by the operation would produce a more firm adhesion of the rectum to the surrounding cellular substance," so as to prevent any return of protrusion. His operation was successful, as Mr. HEAVISIDE's had been; for in each the prolapsus was cured. Mr. HEAVISIDE operated with the ligature, Mr. HEY by excision; either mode gave the same result.

160. Here then we have at once the safest and best principle upon which to operate, for the effectual removal of a prolapsus of the anus, or rectum. The other methods of treatment are palliative; but this may, almost in every instance, be so modified as to effect its purpose with certainty and security.

161. As to the manner of operating, I greatly prefer the ligature: because I have known excision fail, but not the ligature; although I have seen it used by Mr. HEAVISIDE, and had recourse to it myself in very many instances. Previous to operating, the bowels should be emptied by some cooling aperient. Provided, in the operation, any small projection or fold of integuments is found at the verge of the anus, it may be taken up, and will generally answer the purpose: if, on the contrary, the parts around the sphincter are in a perfectly natural state, the tenaculum may be passed through a small extent of the fine integument, at the verge of the anus, carefully avoiding the muscular fibres of the sphincter. The part raised is then to be encircled with a ligature, which being tightened, completes the operation.

162. Where, independent of protrusion of the bowel, the parts surrounding the anus demonstrate extreme laxity, the degree of inflammation required for ensuring the perfect success of the operation will be greater. Here considerable experience and judgment are necessary to determine what the state of constitution will authorise, and what it would be hazardous and unnecessary to adventure.

In some such cases, it is necessary to operate with a degree of boldness; and if one ligature cannot be with tolerable certainty calculated upon as likely to produce a sufficient degree of inflammation, it will be advisable to apply two; one on each side, or otherwise, according to circumstances.

163. It is necessary that the patient be kept quiet for a few days, while the effect of the operation is attended to. If little inflammation takes place, it need not be lessened; if too much, fomentations and the other proper means will moderate its violence.

Where hæmorrhoidal tumours exist, in conjunction with prolapsus ani, the operation that cures the one, if properly performed, removes the other also.

164. From what I have seen, I may venture to assert, that whenever, in early youth, the bowels have been for many days obstinately confined, notwithstanding proper medicines, there will be reason to suspect the existence of intus-susception. This is a fact that cannot be too extensively known

to parents as well as practitioners. Every medical person whatever considers himself competent to direct for what appears to be mere confinement of bowels; and as the number is not small of those who apprehend no ill until either the evil itself, or its fatal consequences, stare them in the face, the above caution may not be without its use.

It is not always a pleasant duty to point out the expediency of taking a second opinion, yet it sometimes is a duty; for in the few cases I have examined of this disease, the patient has, in every instance, died without any suspicion as to the real state of things; while it may be presumed that, had the timely assistance been requested of some surgeon who had seriously applied himself to the subject; life might have been saved, or, at least, some exertion have been made to secure so desirable an object.

165. In some remarks annexed to a case of intus-susception, published some years since, in a truly valuable work*, I suggested, that perhaps the cautious introduction of a large-sized bougie might prove useful in restoring the bowel to its proper situation; but, from one examination I have since made myself, and from another at which I was present, I should now recommend the adoption of other means.

166. The first point is to establish the fact, which, in either of the instances I have seen, could

* Edinburgh Medical and Surgical Journal.

PROLAPSUS ANI, AND INTUS-SUSCEPTION.

at once have been determined by an examination per anum. The next great and essential object is to remove or diminish the constriction, which, in every case I have seen, has existed at that part where the inversion of the external bowel begins. This object must positively be achieved, even though with some risk. For its accomplishment, the warm bath may be tried, and by a proper apparatus, the vapour of warm water may be copiously injected into the bowels. The belly must then be gently, but diligently rubbed, in order to produce diffusion of the vapour. If, in the course of this operation, the mass of displaced bowel is found, by examining per anum, to have retired upwards at all, it may be taken for granted that some part of the intestine is already reduced, a conviction that will afford the best encouragement to perseverance. An additional volume of warm vapour must be rather forcibly injected into the rectum, and the frictions upon the abdomen be repeated, until, by perseverance in the use of these means, the intruded bowel can no longer be felt in the rectum by the finger, or a large-sized elastic catheter carefully passed along the bowel; and, in short, till castor-oil, or some other aperient, has produced a clear passage through the intestinal canal.

167. The above mode of operating, if well managed, may sometimes succeed; but should it fail, something more must be done without loss of time, for I have already stated that the constriction is considerable, and must at all events be relaxed;

for if this is not done, the intestine cannot be returned, and consequently the patient must perish. Should then the vapour of warm water, or warm water itself, aided by the other means, fail, I would not hesitate a moment in trying myself, or recommending to others, the tobacco-fume injection, as by far the most powerful application known, and also as capable of such cautious adoption as to be attended with very little risk; while in fact no other means that I know of, will afford, under these perilous circumstances, the least chance of success.

168. In performing this operation, if the patient be a young child, the tube of the apparatus being secured within the sphincter, one or at the most two compressions of the bellows may be made, and if more inflation be required, it must be completed with common air, care been taken to prevent the escape of the first, while the second is introduced.

If from this operation, followed up by diligent frictions upon the abdomen, some action and rumbling in the bowels in the course of an hour be perceived, without any material impression upon the pulse or skin, one or two more puffs of fume may be ventured upon, as one or two hundred are sometimes borne without inconvenience by a grown person; and in this way, by repeating the same series of operations with precaution, and yet with perseverance, there will be reason to hope for a successful event.

169. I am aware it may be objected, that in some of the few cases that have occurred, neither the nurse nor the practitioner have been able to

make an injection pass. That of course is a difficulty; and if there were no difficulties in the way, the case would be straight forward. The operator must or ought to be a surgeon, prepared to meet and capable of meeting every incident that can occur. A great deal, as relates to the event, will depend on the manner in which the operation is conducted. When the tube of the apparatus is introduced, pressure round the verge of the anus will frequently prevent, or at least impede, the escape of the smoke, until it has produced some effect upon the nearest part of the bowel, after which it will be found very capable of making its own way.

170. The above practical suggestions are applicable to those cases in which there is no outward proof of the existence of the complaint; should the protruded bowel have fallen so low as to appear externally, the event of the case will still depend on the relaxation of the constriction in the superior part of the intestines. Under these circumstances the tube of the fume apparatus must be carefully and effectually inserted between the sphincter ani and the prolapsed bowel, so that the lower part of the rectum may still, as before, be the part inflated. The fume will thus be made to operate where its influence is most wanted, and produce the greatest possible benefit with the least possible risk. Were the injection, on the other hand, made into the orifice of the protruded bowel, instead of being passed up by its side, the fume would go further than is necessary, and its influence on the constriction be

diminished in proportion, while the impression upon the system might prove unpleasant or alarming.

I lately had an opportunity of examining a preparation from the collection of Mr. C. BELL, showing a curious consequence of intus-susception. A young man, in Feb. 1818, after labouring under all the severe symptoms of ileus, with great danger to his life for eleven days, passed by stool a large mass of a solid substance, which proved to be a portion of intestine, partly inverted, measuring nearly thirty inches in length; after which the patient perfectly recovered.

The separated portion of bowel, which appears to be the lower part of the ileum, has evidently been cut off by ulceration at each end, a process that must have taken place at that part where the inversion commenced, in conjunction with the adhesive inflammation that fortunately succeeded in securing the remaining part of the bowels in their newly acquired relations.

Since the above remarks were printed in the former edition, I have met with two very interesting cases, in which, under judicious treatment, aided by the efforts of nature, the patients recovered, after the separation of extensive portions of the bowels strangulated in consequence of intussusception. In one, a girl aged eleven, was attacked, Nov. 20., with pain, distention, and oppression in the bowels; quick pulse, dry skin, and thirst. A purge, an enema, and fomentations, were directed without effect; when, on the 22d, a decoction from half a drachm of tobacco was injected. Syncope, but no evacuation, followed; the pain alleviated, the vomiting continued. On the 23d, purgatives, and the tobacco injection, were repeated; still no evacuation. On the 24th, abdomen greatly inflated; less pain; the medicines remained. 25th, hiccup, and vomiting of fæces, but no proper alvine discharge. Countenance ghastly, pulse quick and feeble, and every sign of approaching dissolution. At seven p. m. a portion of the colon, cœcum, and mesentery, measuring thirteen inches and one quarter; was passed by stool; with much black and fœtid purulent matter, to the amount of six quarts.

From this period the patient progressively recovered, the strength improved, the appetite returned, the pulse became natural, and the bowels regular.

The portion of colon, cœcum, and mesentery, is perfect, and in the possession of Mr. Bowman, who has related the case; to whose promptitude and ability the patient is indebted for her life, and the profession also for a statement full of practical instruction.*

Of the other case, a highly interesting abstract is published by Mr. Renton. A man, after lifting heavy weights, was seized with violent pains in the left side of the abdomen. Various powerful medicines failed in procuring any passage through the bowels, and all the symptoms were approaching fast to a fatal termination, when, on the fourth day

* Edin. Med. Journ. vol. ix.

of the attack, very copious, bloody, and dark-coloured excrementitious stools took place, and the urgent symptoms declined. He continued to improve fourteen days, when he suddenly complained of great distress, and desire to expel something that required all his efforts. From this state he was suddenly relieved by the discharge of eighteen inches of ileum, with a considerable part of the mesentery, which must have been partially separated from the time the passage was restored, fourteen days before.

Much care was necessary to select those articles of diet that agreed with him. Simple and mild food was the best. Animal food, or whatever disagreed, he found reach the seat of irritation in about three hours. Costiveness, induced by the complaint, required the almost daily use of laxatives, as confined bowels always produced attacks of pain, during his convalescence.

Wine, cordials, and malt liquors, were too stimulating, and although weak, he was obliged to avoid them.*

Case 33.

Relaxed and Diseased Rectum.

June 3. 1820. A young woman, of heavy relaxed habit of body, was admitted into St. George's

---

* Edin. Med. Journal, vol. xiii.

Infirmary, with a large and extensive œdematous tumour, at the verge of the anus; and a copious highly fœtid discharge from the cavity of the bowel, as well as from the parts surrounding the opening of the gut. These complaints with an irksome sense of weight, bearing down, and pain in the loins, she had been subject to for the last four years; having commenced soon after her marriage.

She said she had been three months in St. George's Hospital, had used various means and medicines, and was then sent out, the discharge somewhat, but the bearing down and pain in the loins not at all, relieved. She went into service for a few months, when her complaints increasing obliged her to come into the Infirmary.

The disease appeared to be principally, if not entirely, the consequence of extreme relaxation in the inner membrane of the bowel, for there was no particular difficulty or pain in passing a large bougie along the intestine. She said she never had any venereal complaint.

In the treatment, various astringent injections were directed and persevered in for many weeks, and they were certainly very useful. Bark with sulphuric acid were also directed, and were still more essentially conducive to the improvement of her health, and to the lessening the quantity of thin ichorous discharge from within the bowel. Occasionally the fluid excreted was pale and colourless, sometimes yellowish, often of a red tinge, but always of an offensive smell. There was little doubt that the quietude and rest she enjoyed during her stay in the infirmary were also powerful assistants in restoring her health.

August 20. She found her complaint so much relieved, that she left the house to go to service.

Case 34.

Prolapsus of the Rectum.

M. R. complained in October, 1819, of some painful swellings at the verge of the anus. They first appeared during a very severe cold, from sleeping in a damp bed about a twelvemonth before. In September, 1819, she was exposed to much fatigue from very laborious work, when in straining to pass a costive stool a very painful protrusion of the bowel first took place. The prolapsus generally returned whenever she voided a motion, but most extensively when the bowels were confined; although gentle pressure in the horizontal posture always enabled her to return it again.

October 23. I found on examination, a cluster of common hæmorrhoidal tumours, one of the largest of which was secured by a ligature. The parts fomented, the consequent inflammation was moderate. The ligature fell off on the sixth day, and within three weeks the ulcer left by the ligature was healed, and the complaint, to her great comfort, perfectly cured. She was, however, allowed to remain in the house for several weeks afterward, to enable me to determine that the complaint was permanently removed.

Case 35.

Prolapsus of the Rectum.

A. S. aged sixty, was admitted into St. George's Infirmary the beginning of August, 1819. She said that about a twelvemonth before she had a severe disorder in her bowels; violent relaxation, with bearing down, and voiding of blood. During this attack, which continued five weeks, the heavy straining first caused a protrusion of the intestine, which suddenly came down to the extent of several inches, with distressing pain, and a heavy dragging sensation at the loins. She lay down, and pressed it back as well as she could; but her motions, frequent as ten or twenty in the day, always brought it down again.

In the following April she had a troublesome diarrhœa, in which almost every kind of food, with sudden griping pains about the navel, past quickly through the bowels; producing much bearing down, and more prolapsus.

For the first fortnight after her admission into the Infirmary she had frequent thin stools, occasionally tinged with blood. The intestine examined per anum was relaxed, and felt as if the upper had fallen down into the lower part, the whole being thrown into loose folds. On straining to pass a motion, she voided little else than a thin serous fluid, but complained much of her usual dragging and griping pains. The bowel was now down, and in numerous concentric folds or plaits formed a tumour as large as half an orange; it was however easily reduced. She was ordered to take regularly the decoction and tincture of bark; an injection containing eight ounces of the decoction of oak-bark, with one ounce of alum, was also directed to be thrown up twice a day.

August 18. The pains in the back were much relieved, the bowels more regular, and the appetite improved; she even thought that the protrusion of the bowel was much diminished. The medicines were continued.

September 14. The disordered state of the bowels greatly relieved, but after a motion had been passed, I found the prolapsus just the same as ever. A part of the inner membrane of the gut, just within the sphincter, was therefore raised by the tenaculum, with the intention of applying a ligature; but the weak pulpy surface gave way in the attempt. I then passed the instrument through another part of the same membrane, including a small portion of the integument external to the verge of the anus. This was tied firmly, and the patient put to bed.

Little inflammation followed, and the ligature dropped off on the third day. For a few days, her bowels were relaxed, and a trifling degree of protrusion was perceived; her bowels after this acted more regularly, and she had no return whatever of the prolapsus.

Case 86.

Prolapsus Ani.

C. P., aged seventy-eight, had been for two years subject to prolapsus ani, when he was admitted into the St. George's Infirmary, October 4. 1819. The protrusion, which had commenced without any obvious cause, was at first occasional, but soon became more frequent; latterly it seemed to have induced repeated attacks of looseness, a complaint he never had before.

When admitted, his bowels were relaxed. On examination, several small folds of integument were found at the verge of the anus. The prolapsus, when it occurred to its usual extent, included about four inches of the lower end of the gut.

October 5. The largest of the small folds of skin external to the sphincter was included in a ligature. The operation gave but little pain. On the following day, the surrounding parts were very tumid and heated. When he passed a motion the protrusion returned, to about one-fourth its usual quantity. Fomentations were directed to be applied.

October 10. The ligature had fallen off, and the tumefaction quite subsided. He had three motions this day; the verge of the anus was just perceptibly prolapsed on one, but on neither of the other occasions.

December 20. There had not been the least recurrence of the prolapsus, the parts having completely and permanently recovered their tone.

Case 37.

Prolapsus Ani.

Nov. 19. 1820. I was applied to by a lady on the behalf of her little boy, a child of six years old; who for some months had been troubled with a distressing protrusion at the anus, whenever he had a motion, on which occasion he generally had pain, and bleeding. Examining the parts after he had been desired to make some efforts, as in passing a stool, I found a prolapsus apparently the consequence of relaxation and œdema of the highly vascular inner membrane of the bowel; the quantity thus pushed down being in its distended state as large as a cherry. It was returned with facility. On enquiry, it appeared that the bowels, generally regular, were sometimes relaxed.

Nov. 20. With considerable difficulty I was enabled to take up a part of the relaxed margin of the anus, which when tied, formed a tubercle the size of a small garden pea. No apparent inflammation, or only the smallest perceptible redness upon the skin, directly surrounding the ligature, followed. In three days the ligature dropped off, and in four days more the little spot was perfectly healed.

In this instance, the first results of the operation were somewhat different from what I have observed in the adult, although the event was the same.

Dec. 3. All the symptoms were much better than before the operation; the prolapsus, formerly it recurred with every action of the bowels, occasionally several times in the same day, now under regular action of the bowels it appeared only once in three or four days; formerly larger, it was now much smaller. It formerly used to bleed, but this character it permanently lost from the day on which the operation was performed; it used also to remain down till pressed back again; it now returned spontaneously.

Jan. 29. 1821. Upon enquiry, I had the pleasure to hear that the complaint was completely cured; the child for the last six weeks, having had his bowels carefully and watchfully attended to, without the least appearance of any return of the protrusion.

CASE 38.

Prolapsus Ani.

A gentleman, aged forty-three years, consulted me May 10. 1820. His complaint was a continual uneasiness and irritation at the anus. He had been subject to piles, but apprehended the principal complaint was of a distinct nature. Having passed several years in warm latitudes, he had suffered from hepatic inflammation; and since this period had always been attentive to his bowels, which were regular. There was generally notwithstanding a degree of fulness or protrusion at the anus, in passing a motion.

Examining the verge of the anus, I found several relaxed folds of skin, partially loaded with ædema; within these lay a small protruded portion of the inner membrane of the bowel. On enquiring where his uneasiness originated, he said he could touch the spot, and instantly laid his finger upon the projecting point of the inner membrane. By straining a sufficient extent of the lower part of the gut appeared, to prove the existence of prolapsus; not demanding attention from the quantity of the protrusion, nor from the incidental hæmorrhage, so much as from the irritation constantly rendering him unable to attend to business with any comfort, and frequently exposing him to severe pain in walking, riding, or even sitting still. I requested him to take an opening draught that evening; and on the following morning performed the operation.

The tenaculum was passed through the fold of skin on the left side of the anus, upon which lay the relaxed inner membrane, the point of the instrument being so brought out as to include as much of the mucous membrane as possible. A single ligature was applied, and gave very little pain. The following day, he said he felt some pain, and a sense of numbness down the inside of the left thigh. Regarding his habit to be little disposed to inflammatory action, the parts had been merely covered with some cerate upon lint, and he had been requested to keep quiet.

On the third day, the ligature dropped off, the small wound was poulticed for a few days, and then dressed with a weak solution of the nitrate of silver.

On the tenth day, the wound was healed, and he found himself able to sit, or walk, with more comfort than for a long time before the operation. The occasional application of an aluminous lotion, and the daily use of the bidet with cold water, were directed.

On the fourteenth day, I told him there was not the least objection to his returning to business, and took my leave.

In March, 1821, I had the pleasure of hearing that this gentleman had enjoyed good health since the operation; without the least tendency to any return of the complaint.

CASE 39.

Prolapsus Ani; with Abscess.

Sept. 22. 1820. A middle aged gentleman requested me to call upon him. He said he had long been incommoded by what he believed to be the piles; frequently bleeding, but more frequently producing pain and irritation. These circumstances had for two or three years past induced a protrusion of a part of the bowel on going to stool, especially if costive, to which state he was very prone, and had been all his life. He said he had long intended to consult me, and believed he had neglected it too long.

On examination, the tumours were small, but the laxity of parts great. He complained of tenesmus, bearing down, with a sense of heat in one part; but as I could neither perceive redness, tumour, or softness, at any particular point, he was requested to sit for a few minutes on the water-closet, to determine the usual degree of protrusion. The experiment brought down a quantity equal to half a large sized orange; this I returned, and on examining the cavity of the bowel, found it apparently healthy, but relaxed.

I advised him to have the complaint removed by the means I had adopted in other cases; he proposed the operation for the following day, and he was therefore directed an opening draught to be taken at bed-time.

Sept. 23. The medicine, he said, had operated copiously, creating a new kind of irritation and additional pain till just previous to my visit, something appeared to have burst, discharging freely to his great relief. On looking at the part, a small opening was found, and it was clear both to Mr. HEAVISIDE and myself, that the only course was at once to lay open the abscess and sinus, if one existed, and postpone the intended operation; this, therefore, was done, the part was dressed, a warm poultice applied, and the patient put to bed.

Sept. 26. The parts not much inflamed, poured out an excessive quantity of thin, ichorous, offensive discharge. The pulse high, but the spirits very low. Bowels confined and flatulent, bringing down a small part of the lower end of the intestine, in the present weakened state of the sphincter, even while lying down. On examining, found the protrusion was upon the left side of the gut, and that on the left or inverted margin of the bowel were several enlarged and varicose veins, which I touched with a probe; they were partly buried in the substance of the gut, and partly exposed by absorption at certain points of the mucous membrane.

Oct. 2. For the last two days, much improving under the decoction and tincture of bark with the sulphuric acid, after having been several days labouring under a harassing and painful gouty attack in the right great toe; and the skin prone to excessive relaxation, and the whole system the same; a thin ichorous offensive discharge poured out from the bowel and anus, in so excessive a quantity as to require a folded sheet laid under him, changed two or three times a day. Pulse weak, 108, tongue clean and moist, bowels tolerably regular. He was now taking the bark, with port wine, and the most nutritious diet.

Within the last few days I had observed several of the exposed varices, bathed in the unhealthy discharge, gradually lose their consistence, loosen, and finally slough away; leaving the hollow space below purulent, and tolerably healthy. His health, since taking the bark, was so much improved, that he was again able to stand upon his feet without becoming faint.

Oct. 4. Perspiration less excessive; discharge less abundant, and much less offensive.

Oct. 16. Health and strength quiet restored. Pulse down to 80, and strong. The wound from the operation long since healed. Finding the surface from which the varicose veins sloughed out had, from constant exposure to the heat and moisture, been prevented healing, I directed that a saturnine lotion should be applied upon folded lint to the part; which thus became cool, comfortable, and quickly healed. The protruded part of the bowel by degrees shrunk down from the size of a walnut to that of a scarlet bean, gradually assuming the colour and other characters of common integument, from the constant exposure to air. Had I not watched it with continued attention, I could not now have determined it to have been a part of the bowel.

The medicine was now changed for a combination of tonic and aperient, which in a few weeks enabled the bowels to perform their duty with a spontaneous regularity, to which he assured me he had been a stranger for a very many years.

Oct. 25. The protruded part of the bowel perfectly healed, had precisely the same appearance with the other parts of the skin. With the exception of the small portion just mentioned, there was no return of prolapus subsequent to the operation; although, from the partial division of the fibres of the sphincter, the muscle must have been somewhat weakened.

It appears, then, that even the trifling degree of inflammation excited by the operation for fistula, may prove sufficient for the cure of a prolapsus.

Having once felt apprehensive there was contraction of the bowel, he requested me to set his mind at ease upon this point, previous to taking my leave. I therefore first injected a quantity of warm water, a practice I have in many instances found peculiarly convenient, and perfectly effectual for removing the difficulties, of which other practitioners have complained, from the folds into which the bowel is sometimes thrown, obstructing the progress of the instrument; and under this quiet distention, I passed a silver ball an inch in diameter, to the extent of thirteen inches along the canal with the greatest freedom, and without exciting the least sense of uneasiness; proving the rectum to be in every respect sound.

Case 40.

Prolapsus of the Rectum.

A gentleman, aged thirty-eight, came up from the country to consult me for a prolapsus ani, Aug. 16. 1820. He had been subjcet to it for several years; but knew of no cause, his bowels being always tolerably regular. Two years since he had consulted a surgeon of the first eminence, who had directed him to wash with a decoction of oak-bark, and to inject cold water into the bowel before going to stool. The one seemed to relieve the bleeding to which he was subject, the other facilitated the transit of the motion, but neither removed the prolapsus. In July, 1820, a professional friend had performed an operation, by applying a ligature, the object of which was to check hæmorrhage; but it produced no material effect upon the prolapsus. To explain this circumstance, it may be observed, that the operation gave him no pain whatever at the time, and very little afterwards; that he had a motion the next day, without the least pain or uneasiness, and that on the second day the ligature came away.

Aug. 17. I performed the operation, assisted by Mr. Heaviside. In the examination, a little straining brought down the largest mass of prolapsed intestine I had ever seen. It formed a tumour larger than the largest orange. This he said, was the occurrence of every day. The tumour being reduced, the left side of the verge of the anus presented a considerable enlargement, from a relaxed fold of integuments, puffed up with œdema, and replete with enlarged and varicose veins, visible through the skin; and on the margin next the sphincter lay a broad fold of the vascular inner membrane of the bowel. The tenaculum passed through the basis of this tumour a strong ligature was so applied as to include the principal part, together with the fold of the inner membrane. The tightening of the ligature gave considerable pain at first, but by quietude, the reclined position, and the application of a poultice, it was soon rendered easier.

The day after the operation the pain was uniform, and rather severe, but on the following morning (Aug. 19.) it was much better; tongue and skin cool, pulse at its usual standard, 60 in the minute; no disposition to stool, but occasional flatulence.

Aug. 21. Took castor oil, which not operating, he took more: in the course of the day it produced four stools, free and copious, without the least protrusion of the bowel, although, for a long time before the operation, he said he never could go to the water-closet without the part coming down, frequently with much pain, always with bleeding and difficulty in the reduction. The parts were sore, but without any remains of the constant pain that immediately followed the operation.

Aug. 24. Had taken more castor oil, which

had operated twice, without the least protrusion. The ligature fell off in the night; the soft pulp of the slough still remaining attached, the poultice was continued.

Aug. 30. The slough separated, and the wound healing. Having told him he might leave town by the 1st of September, his carriage being adapted for a reclined posture, I gave him a note to his professional attendant in the country, requesting the wound might be dressed with a solution of the arg. nitrat. and the bowels be kept open. He was directed to lay down in his carriage, not from regard to the wound, or the pain that might result, for sitting or walking produced no uneasiness; but having seen the extreme tendency to general relaxation in the parts, I thought it wrong to impose the whole weight and pressure of the abdominal viscera, upon the muscles supporting the anus, so soon after the operation.

Sept. 10. I was acquainted that the wound was perfectly healed, and his health in every respect so perfectly restored, that I could not object to his being out with his gun for three or four hours a day.

On the 24th, I had the pleasure of seeing this gentleman, when he told me he remained perfectly well, though, being very fond of shooting, he had plenty of exercise. The parts examined looked healthy. A tonic draught was directed to be taken twice a day.

Oct. 29. My patient wrote word that, for the

first time, there had been a partial return of the prolapsus; it gave no pain, was attended with no bleeding, and was readily returned. Ordered his medicine to be continued, with castor oil, when required.

Nov. 27. This gentleman called to acquaint me that he was quiet well; that he had on the average walked ten or twelve miles a day, with his gun, without any return of his complaint, and had been on a visit, where he had bathed in the sea, with evident benefit to his health. Violent exercise, or confined bowels, he said, was apt to produce a sense of fulness in the parts. He observed, that now he could scarcely ever perceive even a visible trace of blood in his stools; whereas before the operation, he used always to pass some, and frequently a considerable quantity with his motions; a circumstance which sometimes prevented his accepting the invitations of his friends, from the extreme unpleasantness of seeing the water-closet perpetually soiled with spirits of blood.

CASE 41.

Intus-Susception of the Bowels.

October 13. 1818. I examined the body of a large healthy looking child, who had died the preceding evening, at the age of twelve months, from disordered bowels; and had suckled heartily only an hour previous to his death. For several weeks an apothecary had attended, and directed medicine, at first to remove relaxation, but latterly to relieve costiveness. For a week before his death he suffered constant uneasiness, with so much straining that blood was voided in the fruitless attempts to pass a motion. These symptoms increased, but the child had no more motions, notwithstanding the most active medicines were given, of which some were retained, but most rejected. Repeated attempts were made to procure relief by throwing up an injection; but although the tube was fairly introduced, the mixture would not pass, but returned immediately.

On dissection, I found the bowels inflated. The stomach appeared uncommonly large and vigorous, but touched with the finger it instantly subsided. This arose from an extensive disorganization of its substance, a change in which the stomach had been passive; in colour it was white, as if boiled, and when suspended in water, it was impossible to distinguish the fragments of its coats reduced in different degrees from the bilious and half-digested milk contained within its cavity. This unexpected state was the cousequence of the digestive action having seized upon the viscus itself, almost before it could be said to have lost its vital principle.

On further examination, an intus-susception of the whole extent of the colon was discovered to have been the cause of death. The load of contents within the rectum was very great, and extended downwards quite to the sphincter of the anus. This state of parts had commenced by the lower end of the ileum being pushed down into the larger cavity of the colon; this protrusion having next inverted the head of the colon, and progressively the whole of the remaining part of the intestine, which was thus dragged gradually down through the rectum till it had reached the external opening of the anus.

The present dissection afforded the clearest proof that the fatal constriction exists at the upper extremity of the intus-susception, as already stated. At this part the ileum was received, and another portion of small intestine, the latter having been drawn in by the mesentery attached to the ileum, that had passed down before it.

The displaced parts consequently included the whole of the colon, the cœcum with the appendix cœci, the lower part of the ileum, with a part of another convolution of the small intestine; the inverted head of the colon being the part which must have appeared externally, had the tumour pushed quite through the anus.

The inverted colon, divided longitudinally, exhibited, in a remarkable degree, the occasional effect of strangulation. It was considerably thickened, and of a dark colour, the section demonstrating that these circumstances were owing to a layer of extravasated blood, deposited in the cellular texture between the mucous and muscular coats of the bowel. Some little threads of coagulated blood were still attached to the openings of the overloaded capillary vessels whence the bleeding had taken place, upon the mucous suface of the inverted and strangulated colon, just within the anus.

CHAPTER V.

ON HÆMORRHOIDAL TUMOURS, OR PILES.

Sect. I.

On the Causes.

171. The external integument, or skin, immediately encircling the verge of the anus, is liable to be distended by a deposit of fluids in the cellular membrane, connecting it with the parts beneath. This distension, which may be produced by an effusion either of blood or serous fluid, or both, constitutes the hæmorrhoidal tumour.

172. This kind of tumour, sometimes much inflamed, and often excessively painful, may arise from any irritation in or near the lower part of the rectum: it most commonly depends on some obstruction in the circulation through the hæmorrhoidal veins. Habitual neglect of the bowels, favouring the accumulation of hardened fæces in the rectum; straining to void a confined stool; the pressure of the gravid uterus, or of any preternatural tumour; a sedentary life; sudden and violent exertion; lifting heavy weights; have, in

their turn, been the means of bringing on this disease, and may be considered some of its most frequent causes.

Sect. 2.

On the Symptoms and Appearances.

173. The first appearance of hæmorrhoidal tumour is generally connected with pain and inflammation. The patient usually complains of an uneasy sense of weight and fulness, as well as of heat, about the parts, particularly severe in passing a motion.

174. It has been already observed that these swellings arise either from a deposit of blood, or of serum, beneath the skin. This distinction appears to me worth pointing out, having learned from experience that the means calculated to remove the one kind will not relieve the other.

175. Hæmorrhoidal tumours may be numerous, or otherwise. Sometimes a single swelling only exists; more frequently there are several surrounding the anus.

176. The sanguineous hæmorrhoidal tumour will be opaque, and of a comparatively dark colour, the blood sometimes shining evidently through the skin; it will usually be of more firm consistence, and more slow formation. The serous hæmorrhoidal tumour, on the other hand, will be pale in colour, almost transparent, highly elas-

tic, compressible, and soon produced: the former usually requiring a few days, the latter a few hours only for their production. The sanguineous occur in the strong, the serous are more apt to arise in the weak and irritable. In the sanguineous, the bowels are generally deficient in regularity of action; in the serous this is not so often observed.

177. These complaints, when connected with inflammation, are very painful. The patient can then neither walk, ride, nor sit; the only tolerable state being that of absolute rest in the reclined position. Should he during the continuance of inflammation be obliged to pass a motion, the distress is extreme. With these symptoms there is generally more or less fever-heat and restlessness, now and then delirium.

178. Hæmorrhoidal tumours, when inflamed, are in several respects unfavourably circumstanced. They are surrounded by parts which by their natural warmth tend to keep up, and even increase, local heat; the fulness of the surrounding blood-vessels impedes the circulation, thus aggravating the pain and tension; while the heat and irritation rarely fail to excite frequent and violent spasmodic contraction of the sphincter, almost entirely preventing the return of the blood by the hæmorrhoidal veins that pass up into the bowel between the mucous membrane of the gut and the muscular fibres of the sphincter.

179. Occasional hæmorrhage is in most cases connected with this kind of tumour. Perhaps in the efforts to pass a motion, bleeding comes

on while the parts are inflamed; in this case the blood generally flows from within the anus, though it may occasionally spring from some part of the external swelling. Sometimes the bleeding will first occur and frequently return in the absence of every other symptom; or at least without pain, inflammation, or external tumour.

180. When bleeding has once taken place it may naturally be expected to return, and almost invariably does so; and this return of bleeding, either from its frequency or its extent, uniformly impairs, and sometimes destroys, the constitutional health.

181. The repeated losses of blood progressively lessen the powers of the system, while they introduce habits that, unless attended to, frequently prove of the most serious consequences.

182. When the quantity or volume of the circulating blood is diminished by a part being withdrawn, the loss can be repaired only by the vital powers, whose proper office it is to repair such loss, that there may constantly be kept up a sufficient store for the supply of all the wants and the fulfilment of all the purposes to which the blood is subservient in the animal economy.

183. Hæmorrhage, therefore, as it induces a more rapid waste, incurs at the same time a more prompt reproduction of blood than would otherwise take place; and it must be evident that the circulating system, under the continuance or perhaps increase of this habit, will unavoidably be subjected to great and hazardous

fluctuation, exposing the patient at one time to the distressing and irksome feelings incident to extreme langour and debility, and at another to the more dangerous and suddenly alarming consequences of excessive fulness of blood. (204.)

184. Spasmodic contraction of the sphincter, in the inflammatory or irritable state of hæmorrhoidal swellings, is sometimes a distressing symptom aggravating considerably the sufferings of the patient. Mr. HEAVISIDE has in the course of his practice, in two instances, been consulted, where inflammation taking place in tumours of this description, from exposure to fatigue, the violence of spasm in the sphincter produced complete strangulation, the parts undergoing spontaneous mortification, and the patients obtaining the advantage of a radical cure, without the fatigue of an operation. The possibility of this accident is mentioned by M. LE DRAN.

185. Hæmorrhoidal tumours occasionally occur, in connection either with inflammation, abscess, or fistula in ano; and in several such cases it has appeared to me that they have been the principal exciting cause of all the mischief.

186. In structure, the hæmorrhoidal tumour varies. The serous tumours are in fact little else than the temporary result of œdema, from irritation or inflammation; the sanguineous tumour, on the contrary, is the direct consequence of extravasation of blood.

187. Where a small vessel has ruptured, it usually produces a single tumour at the verge

of the anus, extremely painful, and generally somewhat heated. In one case of this kind, the patient, in passing a confined stool nine days before, felt pain at the side of the anus, which continuing, excited heat and extreme tenderness. A fluid was felt under the skin, with so much pain that I could scarcely persuade him to allow a lancet to be passed into it. This, however, was done, and near an ounce of blood let out. He found immediate and perfect relief, and the cavity was healed within three weeks. In another case a woman complained of a painful swelling at the verge of the anus. Here the tumour was single, and the skin covering it irritable, shining and livid. It appeared to have been produced by a confined stool several days before. The little coagulum of blood was let out, the pain was instantly relieved, and the part readily healed.

188. Where this complaint is the slow result of local debility, or habitual confinement of the bowels, there are generally several unequally-sized tumours round the verge of the anus; should these contain blood, it is most commonly found deposited in separate masses. In examining the structure of a tumour of this kind, the swelling, evidently produced by blood, was neither a varicose vein, nor an effusion from a varicose vein. If it had been the former, the vein might have been seen; if the latter, the effused mass would have been single. The hæmorrhage had evidently proceeded from the capillary vessels in the cellular membrane. The blood had formed cysts in the cellular texture; and the

various tints in the colour of the coagula proved that some had been more recently deposited than others. In some, the same vessel had repeatedly given way, as evinced by the section exposing several concentric laminæ, the external of a brighter colour, the central by gradations darker. The number of coagula in one of these tumours must have been considerable, for upon a single section I counted eighteen; the largest the size of a pea, the rest much smaller.

189. When, from over-distention, the external skin covering a recent coagulum gives way, the vessel may continue to bleed perhaps till the patient is nearly or entirely faint; or should the hæmorrhage occur from within the sphincter, from some one of the veins giving way, the same event may take place; but, in the latter case, the vessel is previously in a weakened and varicose state. The accurate determination of this point has been facilitated by several recent opportunities for prosecuting the enquiry. I once ventured an opinion that where hæmorrhage occurs from within the sphincter, it seems in general more correct to attribute it to some diseased condition of the mucous membrane of the gut, than to relaxation of the coats of any particular vessel. I now, however, know, that in hæmorrhoidal diseases it mostly arises from the rupture of a vein previously enlarged, as I have in several instances ascertained, even where there had never been external tumour.

190. When these veins, situated between the coats of the bowel, become enlarged, they raise

the inner membrane of the gut; this membrane, more exposed than before to pressure from the contents of the intestines, suffers a partial absorption at particular points: these circumstances leave the coats of the vein unsupported, and unavoidably pave the way to subsequent rupture of the vein itself. These facts will be illustrated by the cases.

Sect. 2.

On the Treatment.

191. The relief of the serous hæmorrhoidal tumour is easily accomplished. Absolute rest for a few days, attention to the bowels, and in some cases fomentations, in others cooling lotions to the parts, will generally be all that is necessary.

192. The sanguineous hæmorrhoidal tumour is often attended with much inflammation, requiring, in addition to absolute rest, an active treatment. If the patient is of a full habit, and the parts very turgid and painful, an important step may be the application of some cupping-glasses near the parts. Leeches will occasionally answer the purpose; but if it is required to take away five or six ounces of blood speedily, the operation of cupping is much more certain, as well as more convenient. If necessary, the bleeding may afterwards be encouraged by fomenting with warm water, or a poppy-head decoction. Should the bowels be confined, it

may be prudent to delay for a little the additional disturbance incurred by the passage of a stool perhaps containing hardened fæces, until the symptoms are somewhat relieved; although the procuring a cool and gently relaxed state of bowels is always important, and indeed till this point is gained, little real progress in improvement can be made.

193. Should feverish symptoms demand attention, the proper means will rarely fail to relieve them; saline or antimonial diaphoretics may, if necessary, be added to aperients, and when they have operated satisfactorily there will be no objection to directing an opiate at night, to lessen irritation.

194. Painful spasm of the sphincter may generally be relieved by the continued use of warm fomentations or occasionally by gentle steady pressure upon the tumid parts, by which means part of the blood will be made to pass inward by the hæmorrhoidal veins, relieving the sense of outward fulness.

195. If, during inflammation, bleeding comes on, it will materially assist in unloading the parts, for which reason it should be rather encouraged than repressed, unless the flow is immoderate.

196. Inflammation subdued, the parts subside into a state of comparative quietude; although the passing a motion may still be attended with some degree of pain, or bleeding, or both. In these respects, the health may generally be improved by care to avoid costive-

ness, and by the use of cold water locally, or some astringent application.

197. Where hæmorrhage frequently recurs it generally proceeds from the vessels just within the sphincter, judging from my own experience. That which arises from an external tumour may happen once or twice, but bleedings from the veins within the gut may, and frequently do, return almost daily, for many years.

198. The object which, according to my view of the subject, claims the principal regard in the medical treatment of hæmorrhoidal complaints, is to obtain a regular, easy, and natural action of the bowels, without being under the necessity of having perpetual recourse to purgatives; the consideration of this point, however, would be an anticipation of what I have reserved for the conclusion of these observations, I shall therefore pass on to state what appears to be the best operative surgery in these complaints.

199. Our views must not in the present case be confined to the mere removal of the tumours, they should rather be extended to the adoption of that mode of operating which will most effectually secure the patient from any future return of the disease; and this security can more confidently be expected from the use of the ligature, than by depending on the knife. The ligature also avoids the present risk of serious hæmorrhage, which even the advocates of the knife have admitted is apt to take place from the excision of these tumours, a risk that in

real importance far outweighs any objection yet brought forward against the ligature.

200. In performing the operation, it is not necessary to take up each of the tumours; if there are five or six, the tying of two or three of the largest will generally excite such inflammation as will produce a change in the texture of the remaining parts sufficiently complete to secure the patient from any return of the disease.

201. It has been urged that the ligature is much more painful than the knife, but I have met with only one case in which it was so. It occurred seventeen years since, in a field officer in the army, who had just returned from India. The tumours which I assisted in removing were neither large nor numerous. Only two ligatures were applied, great pain, considerable fever, and some delirium, followed the operation, but usual means for relieving inflammation, assisted by fomentations, brought every thing back in a very few days to a quiet state, without the least delay to the eventual recovery of health, or the effectual cure of the complaint.

202. The practice of some eminent surgeons, who, after having applied the ligature, open the tumour with a lancet, I never adopt; for if the ligature be tied sufficiently tight, the very reason given for the practice falls to the ground, because a part once included in a tight ligature is so effectually cut off from the living body as to be incapable of exciting any sense of pain, or of tension; besides which, the reasons I have already given (131.) in favour of leaving other

tumours to spontaneous decay are equally applicable to those now under consideration.

203. Subsequent to the separation of the ligatures, the fomentations may be laid aside, and the parts may be washed freely with cold water, or kept moist with some cooling lotion, to restore tone, and promote the healing over of the ulcerated points, from which the tumours had been removed.

204. In considering the above operation, we must reflect a little upon the circumstances under which the constitution is placed by its performance. The history of such patients generally informs us that they have been for months, or years, subject to frequent losses of blood the consequences of which upon the system have been already noticed (183.). The tumours removed the patient finds himself no longer subject to bleeding, and usually recovers his strength very quickly. The habit, long accustomed to a drain now cut off, will require some time and some attention, in a medical point of view, before it can accommodate itself to the new order of things. The patient, under these circumstances, should hardly be finally left by his surgeon the moment the operation is performed[*], without even a caution as to any necessary attention to himself in future. On the contrary, the turn of the constitution should, for some little time, be waited for, and watched; and if symptoms arise, indicating local fulness of vessels, they should be met with promptitude. Where this attention is duly shown, the

[*] Case 55.

patient will find himself amply compensated by eventual restoration to a good and even state of health, long unknown to him; while his professional attendant will enjoy the pleasing conviction that naturally arises from every endeavour to do good, added to the consciousness of having proved that the profession of Surgery deserves not to be regarded as an art, but honoured as a science.

Case 42.

Serous Hæmorrhoidal Tumours.

A thin woman, aged forty-six, had been for years subject to severe pains in the back and loins, occasional swellings at the verge of the anus, and an appearance of blood in her stools, whenever confined in her bowels. She said that, when tolerably free from the pain in her back, an extensive irritation, just within the anus, had sometimes appeared to reproduce the external fulness, pain, and swelling. These inconveniences, however, by attention to the bowels and to rest, always went off again.

On the 5th of January, in straining violently, a part of the bowel protruded externally, with much pain, and an irksome complaint of bearing down. By pressure and the recumbent posture it was reduced; and by the next morning she was pretty well recovered. The prolapsus did not return.

January 23. I examined the parts, and found

several small serous hæmorrhoidal tumours, with œdema of the cellular membrane round the verge of the anus. A cold lotion, strongly impregnated with the acetate of lead, was directed to be constantly applied to the parts; the patient was confined to her bed, and the bowels attended to. Under this system the tumours soon disappeared, and in three weeks she was completely relieved from all her complaints; none of which had returned when I enquired after her, four months afterward.

Case.

Serous Hæmorrhoidal Tumours.

Mr. G. a middle-aged gentleman, of a heavy but weak frame, consulted me, Aug. 24. I found him in much pain, extremely depressed in spirits, and incapable of sitting up, from a complaint he had been told was the piles, to which he had been subject for years. With great local irritation and distress, there was so much dread of passing a motion, that, although the bowels were disposed to act regularly, he generally avoided having a stool oftener than once in three or four days. The pulse was quickened, and the tongue furred.

On examining, I found several rather large tumours at the verge of the anus. These tumours were of a pale yellowish colour, almost transparent, and appeared to have arisen from irritation and pressure upon the veins of the rectum.

Strict observance of rest, saturnine lotions, and an occasional aperient, were the means prescribed; which, in a few days, so far relieved him, that he was able to leave not only his bed, but his house also; for he spent his evenings in company. On examining the parts, eight days after I first visited him, neither swelling, heat, nor pain remained. He was, however, desired to take some bark for a few days; subsequent to which, I took my leave.

CASE 44.

Serous Hæmorrhoidal Tumours.

A man, aged forty-eight, complained in June, 1819, of pain in passing his stools, which frequently contained blood; and of a swelling at the fundament from his body coming down, to which infirmity also he said he was subject. On examination, a tumour was found at the verge of the anus. This at first looked somewhat like the protruded bowel, but proved to be several large œdematous, irritable, and painful hæmorrhoidal tumours. By attention to the bowels, by the observance of rest, and by the use of saturnine lotions, the swelling was reduced, and in a week the symptoms were completely relieved; with the exception of some little remaining fulness about the parts.

This poor man had for the last twenty years been subject to an extensive ulceration upon the leg; consequent to which, about three months after the dispersion of the hæmorrhoidal tumours, a large slough formed and separated; during this process the anterior tibial artery suddenly gave way, and he died from hæmorrhage, almost instantaneously. I obtained leave to inspect the body. The lower end of the rectum was removed from the pelvis, and being laid open, was carefully examined. The sphincter of the anus was unusually relaxed, directly above which, the veins of the rectum were seen loaded with blood; for nearly an inch in extent, they were much enlarged and varicose, raising up the mucous membrane considerable above the general surface. When washed with water, the appearance of the bark-coloured veins behind the inner membrane of the bowel afforded a beautiful contrast with the brighter colour of fine arterial ramifications upon its surface.

On considering the appearances of this examination, and particularly those of the blood vessels, it was sufficiently clear, that when bleeding had occurred to any extent from within the sphincter, it could only have been furnished by the giving way of some one of the varicose veins; the largest of which was equal in size to a goose-quill.

Case 45.

Hæmorrhoidal Tumours.

In June, 1820, I was consulted by a most intelligent gentleman, a field-officer in the army, who, having been through all the peninsular campaigns, had suffered in almost every possible way, from fevers continued and intermittent, as well as fluxes; consequent to which several tumours had formed near the anus. These tumours for some months gave extreme pain, but then became easier. For some time, however, a small tender point had made its appearance between these tumours, which, in passing a stool, produced irritation and pain; from this inconvenience he desired to be relieved. He observed that for many years his bowels had never acted without assistance; and as experience had taught him, that the constant use of purgatives was extremely objectionable, he had of late frequently had recourse to injections. A severe bilious headache, also, he said he was subject to, but as he regarded this to be a constitutional circumstance, he looked for no material improvement in this respect.

On examination, I found four hæmorrhoidal tumours; two rather large, though not turgid. On separating them, I perceived a little red tubercle, the projecting point of a protruded fold of the inner membrane of the bowel. Touching this with the end of a probe, he at once recognized it as the cause of all his annoyance. The tumours were subject to some variation, as to size and sensation; but there was no disposition to prolapsus at any time beyond what has been just noticed.

The opinion I gave him was, that the uneasiness of which he complained at the verge of the anus, was very capable of being permanently removed, by the performance of an operation; that the habitual deficiency in the action of the bowels might, I thought, also be corrected by a little attention to medical treatment; and that as for his bilious headache, I was almost convinced, that upon the restoration of the healthy functions of the bowels, the complaint in the head would soon disappear.

For the present, I directed a light tonic, in combination with a gentle aperient; to be taken daily.

July 7. For the last week he had been taking Inf. Cinch. Inf. Gent. C. āā℥fs. Magnes. Sulph. ʒj. in a draught every morning; and said he had not for a great length of time been so well in every respect as now. Much less sense of local fulness; no irregularity or confinement of the bowels; and as for the pain in his head, he did not know when he had been so well as at present.

Aug. 5. I performed the operation, assisted by Mr. HEAVISIDE. The largest tumour, on the left side, was tied first, the ligature including the protruding fold of the inner membrane of the gut. A second ligature was then passed round a tumour on the opposite side of the sphincter, completing the operation. Pain and tumour followed, with troublesome spasms of the sphincter, subsequently quieted by occasioual opiates. In the evening I directed a warm poultice to be applied.

Aug. 6. On changing the poultice, the parts included by the ligatures, were found dark and livid. In my evening visit, I allowed the bidet to be used with warm water, inducing great relief from wind and tension.

Aug. 7. Early this morning, the ligature from the left side was missed; and the tumour had became altogether turgid again at the circle, although the line round it was evident, all behind being alive, all beyond livid and discoloured, although tense.

This accident, which never happened to me before, and which I suspect arose from the influence of the warm bath in relaxing and loosening the knot, was extremely unpleasant. The operation had been attended with more than ordinary pain, and the ligature having slipped, reduced the certainty of success to the chance of 24 or 30 hours' constriction being sufficient to effect the complete destruction of the tumour. Now, although I could myself feel no doubt upon the point, it nevertheless required 14 days' assiduous poulticing, before it separated as an entire firm and hard mass; whereas, the other ligature dropped off with its included soft and putrid tumour, on the ninth day.

Aug. 9. Rather heated and feverish, for which reason I directed some castor oil; it operated three times by the next day, bringing away to his amazement several copious, most offensive, and bilious stools, and that without difficulty or pain, since which time he had found himself much cooler and better.

Subsequent to the separation of the tumours, the ulcerated parts were for a few days dressed with lint, and then with a solution of the nitrate of silver. On the 25th of the month the parts were healed, and all irritation nearly gone. Towards the end of the month, he was able to walk out as well as ever, and took an airing in his carriage. On taking my leave, I requested the tonic draught might be continued for several months, the aperient salt being much diminished in quantity, and generally omitted, being found altogether unnecessary.

In Jan. 1821, I had the pleasure of seeing this gentleman, and had the satisfaction to hear that he had derived every benefit that could have been wished from the operation, as well as from the subsequent medical treatment.

Case 46.

Hæmorrhoidal Tumours.

Sept. 30. 1820. I operated upon a woman aged 45, a patient in St. George's Infirmary, who for several years had been subject to piles. Ligatures were applied to the two largest of the tumours. On the following day her bowels became disordered, for which I directed some gentle aperient medicine to be given. The parts were poulticed; but the pain from the operation was very moderate. The last ligature came away on the seventh day.

Oct. 17. The wounds healed, and the parts quite recovered, she expressed herself extremely thankful, having found herself entirely relieved from the pain and uneasiness she used to feel in passing a motion, and for some time after; adding that she now felt herself more comfortable in regard to health than she had been for many years.

Case 47.

Hæmorrhoidal Tumours.

A strong hard-working woman, aged 59, suffered much inconvenience from an occasional sense of weight, fulness, and swelling at the verge of the anus, in August, 1819. Frequently exposed to great fatigue, the violent bearing down soon produced several distinct and painful tumours; the distress from which was always temporarily relieved by laying down to rest. Now and then, she was subject to disorder and relaxation of bowels; on these occasions, the bearing down, straining, and swelling, were always much aggravated. Under confinement of bowels, she remarked, that the tumours did not come down so low, but the passing a stool was then generally attended with bleeding.

For these complaints she requested to be taken into St. George's Infirmary, Nov. 9. 1820, stating that for the last two months, the constant desire to go to stool, the violent pain and increased swelling, had rendered her almost incapable of standing upright.

Nov. 10. I tied two of the tumours on the left side; the only ones of consequence. An opiate was directed for the evening.

Nov. 14. There was much inflammatory tumour. Some castor oil was given, and operated well.

Nov. 15. Both ligatures came away with the poultice, before the sloughs had entirely separated. By continuing to poultice a few days longer the parts became clean.

Nov. 26. No remaining tumour, the parts quite healed, and all the complaints perfectly gone. Finding herself so well as to be able to stand or walk without pain, she begged to be discharged; it was however deemed prudent to allow her another week's rest; by which time the parts having completely recovered their tone, she was sent out.

Case 48.

Hæmorrhoidal Tumours, with Stricture.

In Sept. 1820, I received a visit from a lady, who stated her complaints to be in the lower part of the bowels, and at the verge of the anus; observing that for their relief, she had already consulted three or four of the most eminent surgeons. She said that several years back, subsequent to a severe complaint in the bowels, she first perceived some little swellings, which were frequently very painful, and that since that period she had occasionally been subject to irritation, and other inconveniences, which she suspected arose from contraction within the bowel.

On examination, I found several small tumours at the verge of the anus; and a stricture to the extent of an inch, just within the sphincter. The contraction was, however, dilatable, and appeared likely to yield to the bougie.

It seemed to me that the first step towards restoring the parts to a healthy state should be the removal of the constant source of irritation kept up by the tumours, and that the next operation would be comparatively easy, in the dilatation of the stricture.

Sept. 13. I tied two of the principal tumours. Irritation and hysterical excitement followed; but soon went off again. An opiate was given at bedtime.

Sept. 17. The bowels having been quiet since the operation, some castor oil was directed, that operated with great relief.

Sept. 18. During the preceding night much annoyed by spasmodic contractions of the sphincter, which, although quiet while awake, never failed to disturb her, the very moment of dropping off to sleep; notwithstanding the opiate, which was repeated every night.

Sept. 19. I was acquainted that an irritation anterior to the passage of the bowel, which, from frequency and severity had for many months been productive of great distress, had returned but once since the operation, and then only to a very trifling degree.

Sept. 20. The ligatures came away with the poultice, leaving a clean and healthy surface.

Oct. 12. Some interval allowed to pass subsequent to the healing of the wound, an elastic gum bougie, three-eighths of an inch diameter, was passed through the stricture, and kept there five minutes, without pain. She said she found herself greatly relieved in every respect, by the late operation.

Nov. 6. Having successively increased the diameter of the bougie, until one of full size passed with ease, and finding also that the passage of the motions had ceased to excite the least sense of uneasiness, this lady took her leave of me, preparatory to visiting the country.

During the above attendance, upon repeated complaints of the want of regular action of the bowels, as well as of dislike to the constant use of purgatives, I for some weeks directed medicines upon the principle laid down in the concluding part of these observations, with perfect success; and consequently very much to the satisfaction of my patient.

Case 49.

Hæmorrhoidal Tumours.

Aug. 30. 1820. A middle-aged gentleman called upon me, who stated that from confinement of bowels, during a long journey through Italy, some painful tumours formed within the verge of the anus; and that in April last, a surgeon, a friend of his, had performed an operation, and with scissars had cut off three hæmorrhoids from the inner surface of the bowel, telling him he would engage that he would never be troubled with that complaint again. Upon this point he was desirous of hearing my opinion.

On examination, I found there had been tumours, but that now there were none. The cavity of the bowel was healthy, but the parts within, and at the verge of the anus, much disposed to relaxation and fulness. As to my opinion, I acquainted him that I considered it of the first importance to keep up regular action in the bowels, to ensure as far as possible the continuance of his present health; but that as to any absolute security from future return of the complaint, I could not express so confident an opinion as his friend had done, although by attention and care, he might perhaps avoid it.

CASE 50.

Ulcerated Hæmorrhoidal Tumours.

Nov. 14. 1820. I assisted Mr. HEAVISIDE in the examination of a stout middle-aged gentleman, in whom there was reason to suspect the existence of a fistula; as a constant, and as it was stated, sometimes a considerable discharge could not otherwise be well accounted for. Mr. HEAVISIDE had operated once on this gentleman for fistula fourteen years before, from which operation he quickly recovered.

We found an immense cluster of what had originally been a succession of hæmorrhoidal tumours, some sanguineous, others serous; but from age and other circumstances, they were now rendered flat and thin, having the appearance of so many uneven plaits or folds of thin skin. In some of these, varicose veins, in others, little masses of effused and coagulated blood, were visible through the fine skin. They were so numerous, as to render the examination of the parts very difficult. After a diligent search, neither sinus nor opening into any cavity could be detected; but after much trouble, the daily appearance of matter upon the linen was explained, by finding, at the margin of the anus, towards the perineum, that the basis of one of the tumours had ulcerated to the extent of a sixpence. Upon enquiry where the pain was felt, and whence he supposed the discharge to proceed, he placed his finger exactly on the spot.

Taking a West-India constitution into the account, it was deemed advisable to direct a gentle cooling and astringent lotion, to be applied daily upon lint, keeping the parts quiet, and the bowels open; by these means the discharge was soon diminished, and the complaint eventually removed.

Case 51.

Hæmorrhoidal Disease.

N. R. aged fifty-two, was admitted into the St. George's Infirmary, April 1. 1819. He stated that about ten years back he had been subject to frequent bleeding from the rectum; the blood flowing freely, whether the bowels were neglected or attended to. These symptoms had continued some months, when several painful tumours formed at the verge of the anus, which for many weeks continued to annoy him with acute and shooting pains. For their removal he was advised by an acquaintance to expose the parts to the acrid fumes of burning sulphur. The experiment produced intense pain, and some inflammation. The tumours, which before were full, dry, and smooth, now became cracked, moist, and shrivelled, oozing out a serous fluid.

Fom this time he remained nearly free from the complaint till a twelvemonth since, when from exposure to good living and hard work, the bleedings returned, and became frequent and considerable. In place of the former tumours, he was now inconvenienced by some excrescences, that excited much irritation, excreting an offensive serous moisture. A saturnine lotion was applied for two months, without much diminishing the discharge, although it relieved the heat and lessened the irritation.

April 4. 1819. These excrescences were removed. As the patient had latterly complained much of weakness, and even occasional prolapsus, it was considered advisable to try whether the largest of the tumours would bear the ligature, in expectation, that if it were practicable, the tone of the parts might be thus improved. A ligature was placed round the basis of the largest, but on tightening it the substance of the excrescence was pinched out of its place, leaving its thin covering of skin behind. They were therefore separately snipped off, with a pair of scissars.

In the early part of May he took cold, and was much disordered in his bowels; for this disorder he was seen by the physician; the complaint, however, increased, a colliquative diarrhœa followed; and on the 12th of the month he died.

On examination, the lower end of the rectum was found enlarged, and its coats thickened. The bowel laid open, its inner membrane appeared thickened, pulpy, and thrown into large loose folds, among which were found little masses of a transparent whitish jelly. At the posterior part of the rectum, just within the sphincter, the bowel was for the space of a shilling ulcerated, with a thickened margin, overhanging the basis. The surface of the ulcer was purulent, with numerous small brown points, that with a glass appeared to be sloughing granulations.

Externally, by a small opening, a probe found its way into a sinus behind the muscular band of the sphincter, and came out upon the ulcerated surface of the bowel. The sinus passed through a little abscess that had formed in the cellular membrane. At the superior part of the ulcer, within the rectum, there was also a little opening, leading higher up into another abscess, not larger than a pea, seated in the cellular membrane of the gut.

Several tumid and varicose veins were seen through the inner membrane of the bowel, just within the sphincter, the varices being nearly equal in magnitude to those observed in another instance.* Some of these veins were excessively enlarged, and one had ruptured into the cellular membrane, the extravasated blood forming a coagulum the size of a large grape.

CASE 52.

Sanguineous Hæmorrhoidal Tumours.

In September, 1813, I was consulted by a lady, who had been for some time inconvenienced by a complaint extremely painful in walking, or even sitting down; more particularly when her bowels were confined.

On examination I found several hæmorrhoidal swellings; as the bowels required no previous attention, two of the largest tumours were immediately tied. Considerable pain and inflammation followed, with an unpleasant irritation at the neck of the bladder, and a mucous dis-

* Case 56.

charge from the vagina. Fomentations, however, with an opiate at night, very soon removed these symptoms, and on the fourth day the one, on the seventh the other ligature came away. A cooling lotion applied to the parts for a week longer completed her perfect recovery; since which time this lady has enjoyed good health, and has no tendency to any return of her complaint.

Case 53.

Sanguineous Hæmorrhoidal Tumours.

Mrs. B. aged thirty-four, applied to me, April 28. 1813, on account of some hæmorrhoidal tumours. She said they had existed for several years, but had of late produced much distress, being occasionally attended with severe pain, and sometimes inflammation. There were, in this case, five distinct tumours, but I found it sufficient to tie three of the largest. The inflammation that followed was moderate, and was much relieved by fomentations. The last ligature came away on the fifth day; and, within three weeks from the operation, the parts had entirely recovered themselves, the patient being restored to perfect health.

Case 54.

Sanguineous Hæmorrhoidal Tumours.

October, 1815, I operated upon Mr. M. a gentleman aged thirty-four. The tumours, of the sanguineous kind, had occasionally produced much pain and distress, and were attended with bleeding from within the anus. I applied only two ligatures, the last of which came away on the fifth day. In a few days more he felt himself mending apace, and within a fortnight after the operation the parts were perfectly healed; since which time he has enjoyed good health.

Case 55.

Sanguineous Hæmorrhoidal Tumours.

A gentleman, in the thirty-sixth year of his age, requested my opinion in January, 1819, upon some swellings at the verge of the anus. He said, that about four years back he had consulted a surgeon of the first eminence at the east end of the town, for the same complaints, who had given him no opinion, but had performed an operation upon him by snipping away a small part of the projecting fold of the inner membrane of the bowel, and then cutting open one of the largest of the tumours, desiring him to keep quiet, and to have a poultice applied. As, to his surprise, he saw no more of his surgeon, and had received no direction as to management, he requested his apothecary to look after him. He soon recovered from the operation the object of which, he supposed, had been to remove the tumours themselves, as well as the frequent bleedings from the rectum, to which he had for some years been subject.

Subsequent to the operation, he found that the appearance of blood in his stools was less frequent; but his bowels, naturally disposed to costiveness, now became more confined than ever. He also became subject to a frequent attack of a new kind, a heaviness and swimming in the head, sometimes to an alarming extent, for which his physician had of late repeatedly directed him to lose blood by cupping. For these complaints he consulted me, not concealing his anxiety to avoid, if possible, the necessity for cupping, as he very justly considered it a bad habit, and of dangerous tendency. His stools, at this time, were always mixed with blood, of which he had lost, during the last fortnight, as much as from one to four table-spoonfuls each day, dependent on the state of his bowels. I examined the parts, and finding the tumours themselves did not require any immediate attention, it appeared to me that the plan most likely to serve him was to direct medicines, the object of which should be to establish a regular, easy, and gently relaxed state of the bowels, not by incessantly exciting their languid powers by purgatives, but by endeavouring to restore them to their natural tone, thus enabling them to perform their functions punctually and perfectly, without the assistance of aperients.

As to the particulars of the treatment it is only necessary at present to say it succeeded, and that, in two months, he not only found himself comfortable and regular in his bowels, unsolicited by medicine, and unassisted by any other means; but had lost all traces of blood in his stools. The complaint in his head also was relieved, and eventually left him entirely under the measures that were adopted; a circumstance that afforded both himself and his family infinite comfort.

In the following summer this gentleman visited Brighton; on his return to town he called and assured me he had not passed a season in such good health, either as related to regularity of bowels, or freedom from any unpleasant sensation in his head for many years; he also observed, that he had neither been incommoded by bleeding, pain, or external swelling.

Case 56.

Varicose Hæmorrhiodal Veins.

May 20. 1817. I opened the body of R. P., aged sixty-six. His complaints had been a complicated disease of the urinary organs; and the circumstance of the water having passed by the rectum for a long time before his death, induced me to examine the intestine with peculiar care.

The veins in the rectum, just above the sphincter, formed a considerable varicose cluster. In two points, but particularly in one, an angle of one of the enlarged vessels projected beyond the rest, towards the cavity of the bowel. At these points, for an oval space near an eighth of an inch in length, the dark-coloured blood within the veins was so clearly apparent, that it might almost have been doubted whether there was any substance at all interposed between it and the eye. On a minute examination it appeared that at these points the coats of the vein and the internal membrane of the bowel were undergoing a progressive absorption, consequent to which any trifling circumstance might have produced a rupture of the thin film that remained between the venal blood and the cavity of the gut. From the appearance of these points it was evident the change was progressive and slow. Observed under a magnifying glass, the blood was most evident, and the absorption of its covering membranes consequently most nearly complete in the centre, from which to the circumference the discolouration became less perceptible till it quite disappeared.

This dissection clearly explained the principle on which a varicose vein gives way in the rectum; proving that it may, and probably does, occur, whenever such vessel is so raised beyond the general surface as to be particularly exposed to pressure from the transmission of indurated contents through the bowels, such pressure operating by exciting irritation, and absorption, as its eventual consequence.

CHAPTER VI.

ON FISTULA IN ANO.

Sect. 1.

On the Causes of the Disease.

205. The cellular and adipose substance surrounding the verge of the anus, in common with the same texture elsewhere, is subject to inflammation and abcess. This may arise here from any of those causes known to produce similar changes in other parts of the body;—any external violence; any irritation within, or near the extremity of the rectum; and particularly that excitement sometimes consequent to fever. A severe cold frequently operates as a cause; excessive fatigue also has, in some instances, apparently been the means of inducing inflammation and abscess near the anus.

206. The causes productive of fistula in ano, will, as to their mode of operation, very much depend on the habits and health of the patient. Where the health is bad, or, where the constitution is highly disposed to scrofulous action, I have known the most trivial circumstances bring on a train of ill consequences of so serious a discrip-

tion, as to baffle the best efforts of surgery*, when, however, the habit being sound, the case is early attended to, the most violent attack, or most alarming accident, frequently proves perfectly manageable, terminating well beyond any reasonable expectation.

Sect. 2.

On the Symptoms and Appearances.

207. The existance of a sinus, or, what has been termed a fistula in ano, has been supposed to indicate in every case a depraved habit, and in particular an unhealthy condition of the parts affected. This, however, is by no means true. The mere production of a sinus is a circumstance dependent upon a general principle that should never be lost sight of by the practical surgeon, being as frequently applicable to other kinds of abscess, as to that now under consideration. Observation evinces that, wherever an abscess forms in cellular membrane, the matter is apt to burrow, where it meets least resistance; in other words, it is disposed to extend the limits of the abscess in whatever direction the cellular membrane is most relaxed: upon this principal the matter frequently makes its way to some extent along the rectum, penetrating between the coats of the bowel, and forming a narrow sinus, or fistula.

* Case 62.

208. The early stage of the inflammatory attack, in the young and healthy, usually presents a circumscribed prominent tumour, heated, red, and painful; with quickened pulse, hot skin, thirst, and white tongue, dependant on constitutional sympathy. Under neglect, or mismanagement, this re-action of the system will sometimes occasion high fever, and delirium.

209. Phlegmonous or healthy inflammation in these parts would, perhaps, generally terminate in suppuration, were nothing done for its relief; but inflammatory action so readily extends itself, and the various organs in the intermediate vicinity are so delicate in their structure, and so important in their functions, that decision is no less necessary than discrimination at the onset of the attack, to ensure as far as possible, a favourable event.

In no case that I know of is neglected inflammation productive of more permanently distressing consequences to the patient, than in the present complaint; although this is one of the many truths the real importance of which is seldom duly appreciated till it is learned by painful experience.

210. In some instances a considerable degree of constitutional excitement may attend local tumour, more extensive, and less distinctly circumscribed than the above, the dull red colour, and the less elastic feel of the parts exhibiting the characters of erysipelas. There may, in this case, be more disease of cellular membrane, but the suppuration will be less perfect, and less plentiful, than in phlegmonous inflammation.

211. Occasionally the inflamed parts may assume a lurid and dusky colour, and although harder than natural, there shall be less tension than belongs either to phlegmon or erysipelas; the pulse being full and hard, the thirst great, and the restlessness fatiguing. In this state of things, unless, the patient is soon relieved by medicine, the pulse, strength, and spirits, all give way together, and since to an alarming extent. Should matter be formed, it is, as Mr. Pott has well observed, small in quantity, and bad in quality, the cellular membrane being extensively sloughy and gangrenous. This is the " suppuration gangreneuse" of the French authors.

212. Some degree of irritation at the neck of the bladder generally attends the formation of matter in its neighbourhood. This may excite uneasiness in making water, or anxiety to avoid the urine, or produce so much spasm, as to bring on a total retention of urine. From the same cause may arise temporary irritation, or painful fulness at the lower part of the rectum, inducing an irksome bearing down, hæmorrhoidal tumours, frequently confinement, but now and then relaxation of the bowels.

213. When an abscess is formed, a part of the surface becoming softer than the rest, the skin usually gives way, allowing the escape of the contents. Sometimes, however, I have found the first discharge arise from the sinus having burst into the intestine.* The most common state presents a single external opening near the anus, generally

Case 11.

with a sinus passing up by the side of the bowel; in other cases there is one opening from the abscess externally, and another by the sinus into the cavity of the intestine.

214. The late Mr. POTT, in his excellent treatise upon this subject, has stated that fistulous complaints do not very unfrequently stand upon a venereal basis; and so far as the existence of sinuses communicating with the neck of the bladder, and also with stricture in the urethra, may confirm such opinion, I have myself, in repeated and frequent instances, had the care of cases decidedly of venereal origin.

215. The appearances that occur in the examination of a sinus, or fistula in ano, are usually confined to an ulcerated space, more or less extensive, in the adipose membrane near the anus, connected with a narrow canal or sinus, admitting a probe to pass for some extent upwards between the coats of the bowel; communicating with the cavity of the intestine, or not as it may happen. The parietes of the abscess in healthy inflammation demonstrate the induration consequent to effusion of coagulable lymph into the cellular texture surrounding the cyst; the same appearance being to a certain degree generally perceptible along the line of the sinus immediately connected with the intestine.

216. In erysipelatous inflammation, and especially in the gangrenous suppuration, the cellular membrane exhibits the principal traces of disease; in the former case this texture is usually inflamed, and disposed to slough, in the lat-

ter it is found more extensively sloughy and gangrenous.

217. Those cases in which abscess takes place within the pelvis, or high up towards the loins, generally derive their formidable character from the circumstances under which matter is deposited, as it is almost invariably found to have injured, or destroyed, some part of one or other of the bones of the pelvis; and even the importance of these cases, is, upon enquiry, generally found to have been derived from long neglect on the part of the patient. In one case of diseased hip, connected with a sinus that passed over the tuberosity of the ischium, I found, on dissection, three or four fragments of the bone carious, separated, and black; one of the fragments had partly made itself a passage out through the soft parts. I have seen several other cases nearly similar; but in examining one where an abscess behind the rectum had formed within the sacrum, I found the peritoneum thickened, sloughy, and separated from nearly the whole concave surface of the bone; which was consequently bare, and black as charcoal; the open texture of the necrosed bone being saturated with a dark-coloured offensive purulent fluid.

SECT. 8.

On the Treatment.

218. IN the treatment of phlegmonous inflammation near the anus, should the local heat, pain,

and tumour, be considerable, we must sometimes have recourse to blood-letting. If the habit and pulse are full, as well as disturbed, a vein may be opened in the arm; in other cases it will be sufficient to take away a much smaller quantity near the seat of the affection by leeches, or cupping. This measure may occasionally be expedient, not so much to prevent suppuration, as for the more important purposes of moderating the extent of inflammatory action, and promoting the favourable operation of the other means of relief.

219. The assiduous use of fomentations also is to be directed, and continued till the abscess is formed, and its contents discharged.

220. The central part of the tumour becoming soft, the external skin may be permitted to become thin, before it is opened with a lancet; when this opening is made, it must be prevented from closing directly, by the insertion of a few threads of lint. After the abscess is opened, the parts may still be fomented for a few days, till all the inflammation, and most of the surrounding hardness, have subsided. Under these circumstances the cavity of the abscess, provided the discharge is healthy, will contract apace, and be very soon healed.

221. Abscess near the anus will frequently heal, even under total neglect; but it generally happens, under these circumstances, that the parts do not entirely recover their healthy feelings, but on the contrary, remain subject to permanent uneasiness and irritation.*

* Case 56.

222. If the abscess does not heal readily, or should the flow of matter be greater in quantity, or worse in quality, than it ought to be, a probe gently introduced, will easily determine whether a sinus exists, either towards the bowel, or in any other direction.

Should febrile symptoms be urgent, they may be relieved by some of the means already suggested (34.), without interfering with the other objects, which must, in the present case, be held in view.

223. In the second kind, or erysipelatous inflammation, bleeding is but seldom proper, neither will the patient bear the free adoption of other evacuations. The occasional use of gentle aperients, however, will be essentially useful. Warm and emollient fomentations must be applied, and when suppuration commences, although it may be imperfectly established, it will be right to make an opening, which, by allowing the escape of matter, will diminish the risk of further extension of disease in the cellular membrane.

224. In the third kind of inflammation, hot spirituous fomentations must be applied; free incisions be made into the diseased parts, and recourse be immediately had to medicines. The patient should be directed the cinchona, in combination with other tonics and opiates, so adminsistered as to afford the most effectual aid in restoring a broken constitution.

225. Where, from the formation of abscess, irritation, or spasm takes place at the neck of the bladder, opiates, and a free use of mucilagin-

FISTULA IN ANO.   211

ous decoctions, will generally procure relief. When this affection goes on to retention of urine, anodyne relaxation must still be the leading principle in treatment, aided by evacuations from the bowels, and also by blood-letting, together with fomentations, followed by an emollient and opiate glyster.

226. Irritation excited in the rectum, may be relieved by the gentle operation of some mild aperient; or the exhibition of a warm emollient injection. Should obstinate costiveness occur, from the accumulation of hardened fæces, no time must be lost in procuring relief; for while this state continues, every symptom will be aggravated. Repeated aperients, the injection of laxative glysters, in some cases assisted by the abstraction of blood, will be the proper means; neither must they be laid aside till there is reason to feel assured that the bowels are cleansed, and the system consequently relieved, from that which experience teaches, may otherwise prove a source of infinite irritation, and many distressing symptoms.

227. When abscess is formed, and its contents have been discharged, it will in general be proper to ascertain whether a sinus exists or not. If such be found, the sooner it is divided the better. In effecting this division, every surgeon who duly regards his patient's feelings, and his own character, will prefer that mode of operating, which accomplishes its object with the least pain, the least delay, and the greatest certainty of a successful event; and this mode is most cer-

tainly that in which the division is made with the probe-pointed bistoury.

228. In performing the operation for fistula in ano, a probe first passed into the sinus traces its direction and extent along the side of the gut. The fore-finger of the other hand, previously oiled, is then passed through the sphincter, so as to feel distinctly the point of the probe; this being withdrawn, the bistoury is to be lightly and gently introduced in its place, till the point of the instrument in the sinus is made to press against that of the finger in the rectum. In this stage of the operation, should no direct opening be found from the sinus to the bowel, the least additional pressure of the point of the bistoury against the finger may be made to bring them into actual contact. The point of the finger now becoming a guide to the bistoury, presses the instrument on before it, so that while the finger is gradually withdrawn, the bistoury is made to cut its way out, and the operation is finished.

229. The parts are to be lightly dressed with a narrow slip of fine lint, carefully introduced along the course of the sinus, in such manner as to prevent the union or contact of the recently divided parts; for unless this is prevented, the operation may fail.

230. Where the abscess is large, or the habit unsound, sinuses are frequently found passing in various directions beneath the integuments. These must be severally laid open, and regularly dressed in such manner as to give a gentle sti-

mulus to the parts, and prevent any lodgment of matter.

231. In the many operations of this kind I have either performed myself, or seen performed by others, some few have been attended with a rather considerable loss of blood; but I have never known an instance in which there was the least real difficulty in restraining the hæmorrhage. The most vexatious case that has ever occurred to me with its treatment, will be mentioned presently.*

282. Occasionally, though rarely, the disease is not capable of cure by the above means. Where the constitution is unhealthy, whether from age, debauchery, or other cause, difficulties may arise. In one case, as fast as the divided sinuses heal, others form, and are unexpectedly discovered; in another, the sinuses, when laid open, will not heal, pouring out, for a tedious length of time, a thin offensive discharge. Under these circumstances recourse must be had to medicine, with a view to improve the tone, increase the strength, and diminish the irritability of the system. In these cases, I have sometimes found change of air effect that improvement of constitution which medicine had failed in accomplishing.

283. It may happen that, either from inattention or ill health, the constitution may be so reduced as to render the immediate performance of the operation unadviseable; medicine must be directed, and as the appetite becomes establish-

* Case 61.

ed, and the strength restored, the state of the local complaint will be observed to improve, till at length the parts assume the appearances of health, previous to which an operation would be at least useless, if it had no worse tendency.*

234. Now and then it may be difficult to determine accurately on the state of constitution, till after the operation; when the patient shall rapidly decline into a state of unexpected laxity and exhaustion, requiring the most vigilant, active, and persevering attention, to ward off a threatened ill event.†

Case 57.

On Fistula in Ano.

A. P. aged forty-three, applied to me, September 15. 1819. For two months she had experienced a distressing uneasiness and bearing down, when moving about, particularly upon sitting down. There was also a sense of heat, with a pain which she thought proceeded from a swelling forming within the bowel. These symptoms were greatly aggravating upon going to stool.

In the course of a few days, inflammation was evident externally, with tumour and extreme pain in the right side of the sphincter. Poultices were applied, and in eight days she was relieved

* Case 62.   † Case 39.

by the bursting of the abscess, which discharged abundantly.

The first abscess broke on the 26th of August, but a second inflammation succeeded, and after several days' severe pain some matter escaped by the former opening, September 13th. On the 15th I first visited her, and on examination found a sinus running to the extent of three inches between the coats of the rectum. At her own request I immediately introduced a bistoury, and divided the sinus. The operation was attended with little bleeding, and less pain. Under the usual treatment she went on so well, that on the 23d of the month she was walking about the room, without the least pain or tenderness; and on the 29th, (the 15th after the operation,) I found that for several days there had been no trace of discharge; on examining, the sinus was found perfectly healed, the cavity of the rectum being cool, quiet, and in its natural state.

CASE 58.

Fistula in Ano.

J. Davidson, aged thirty-six, came into the St. George's Infirmary, August 19. 1818, with a purulent discharge, consequent to abscess at the verge of the anus. On examination, a fistula, extending near two inches along the side of the gut, was discovered and divided. No material bleeding followed, nor any other particular circumstance either at the time or subsequent to the operation; which enabled the patient to leave the infirmary, perfectly cured of his complaint, on the 7th of October following.

Case 59.

Fistula in Ano.

A coachman, aged fifty, applied to the St. George's Infirmary, February 11. 1820. Many years subject to piles, he was attacked on the 2d instant with pain at the verge and within the sphincter of the anus, which obliged him to keep his bed. A considerable tumour had formed, extremely painful to the touch within the bowel. On the 8th, there was more softness and less heat in the swelling, to which fomentations were continually applied. On the following day it broke, and gave him relief by a free discharge. On the 11th, I found a fistula passing for an inch along the side of the gut, which I divided without any bleeding or much pain. The sinus did not open into the bowel. Within three weeks it was perfectly healed; and the man, perfectly recovered, returned to his work.

Case 65.

Abscess in Ano.

A gentleman came to town to me October 10. 1820, complaining of frequent uneasy sensations at the verge of the anus; in a spot where there had been a small abscess two or three years before, which after some time healed spontaneously. He observed that ever since, he had been subject to pain or uneasiness in the part; after fatigue or exercise. The rectum examined, was healthy, but in a lateral point within the sphincter, he said he could feel the irritable spot, as also externally where a little apparent thickening existed.

I told him, that most probably he would be liable to return of inflammation and abscess from the first accidental cause, and that then it might be more easy to cure his complaint, and effectually prevent its return, then at present; and that as to the peculiarity of his sensations they appeared to depend on the parts not being yet restored to a state of perfect health.

Case 61.

Fistula in Ano.

A man, aged thirty-two, was admitted into the St. George's Infirmary, with abscess near the fundament. On examining, I found an extensive sinus, between the coats of the bowel. As the parts were healthy, and the poor man desirous of relief, I performed the operation immediately, laying open the whole length of the sinus, and dressing the parts in the usual manner. In the course of the evening, I was requested to visit him, and found he had been bleeding for the last hour, and from the state of the clothes it appeared that he had lost near a pint of blood. His pulse was much softer than natural. I therefore desired the whole of the bed-clothes to be thrown aside, and that he might be laid on his face, with his head lower than the rest of his body, his hips being raised upon some bolsters and pillows. The parts, thus exposed to a current of fresh cool air, were kept covered by a succession of clothes dripping wet from a pail of cold water, and changed every five minutes. These means, which immediately arrested the hæmorrhage, were however directed to be continued for a few hours, after which a sheet was thrown over him, and on the following morning he was allowed to resume a comfortable position in bed. This man was discharged, perfectly cured, within three weeks after the operation.

Case 62.

Fistula in Ano.

In the year 1817, a poor man was admitted, at the age of sixty-three, into the St. George's Infirmary. His complaint had originated in an abscess that had formed about seven weeks before, near the anus. The integuments were rather extensively separated from the parts beneath, the ulcerated cavity secreting an excessive quantity of unhealthy and fœtid purulent matter. The low pulse, extreme debility, and great emaciation, were so many proofs of the injury already sustained by a shattered constitution. A probe readily found a sinus passing along the side of the rectum for more than three inches within the sphincter.

The state of the case was such as to forbid the performance of any operation, till by attention to diet and medicine, the ill condition of his habit might be improved, and his strength in some degree restored. With this view, every attention was paid to the daily regulation of his diet, and the same regard shown in the adjustment of his medical treatment; but notwithstanding every exertion made for his recovery, he lost ground; his appetite and strength continued to decrease, and about a month after his admission into the house, he died.

Case 63.

Scrophulous Fistula, in Ano.

A married woman under thirty, applied to me for assistance, for fistula. On examination, a sinus presented itself within an inch of the anus; it was a gaping smooth orifice, with hardened edges. In the middle of the nates, I could insert three fingers into the orifice, and my middle finger could feel bands contracting the passage; but the finger could be passed under the illium, close upon the bone. Another course branched up by the side of the cleft of the nates towards the sacrum; added to these there were two blind passages of sinuous course running along the side of the rectum, the left one of which nearly made a communication with the gut, two inches or more within it.

On looking at her countenance it was truly scrophulous, fair, red, and white, with prominent sparkling eyes, large pupils, but the maxillary protuberance of the left cheek certainly greater than that of the right.

Attention was paid to the constitutional symptoms, and her health improved. She stated, that the first consequence of her illness was a large tumour, which was opened in its deep seat. This had discharged copiously, bringing her health into great jeopardy, and threatening a phthisical termination in a highly nervous irritable habit. The very proposal of an operation destroyed the appetite for several days, inducing diarrhœa. In jections had had a fair trial, no chance of recovery offered, unless by mending the habit; assisting at the same time the local condition of the parts. Pressure, with lead and bandage, was for some time persevered in, with little change of action. I therefore introduced a bistoury, cutting asunder the bands in the passage, and pressure was again resorted to, but still the healthy process was not much advanced. A curved rectum trocar was next introduced at the nates, conducted up under the illium, pushed out through the fascia lata on the external side of the thigh, a seaton inserted, and the sinuses near the gut divided in their full extent.

The seton was retained till the moving it produced bleeding, by the friction, when it was withdrawn. From May 7 to August 10 her condition was so much mended, that she followed her household occupations and came to me twice, improving much in every respect, a distance of three miles; when I conceived that time alone would complete her cure, especially as the catamenia had returned. I requested to see her occasionally, but this she neglected, till within a week I was again sent for. She said she had taken cold; her thigh had gathered and discharged copiously, a highly fœtid matter. The sinuses still existed, though much contracted, secreting a gleety lymph; but the skin was thickened and the cellular membrane with a puffy tumour, upon a spot or two of which a little fluctuation might be perceived. She was now placed under a course of sarsaparilla, and liquor potassæ; with diligent frictions of camphorated mercurial ointment.

CHAPTER VII.

ON THE HÆMORRHOIDAL EXCRESCENCE.

Sect. 1.

On the Causes of the Disease.

235. The hæmorrhoidal excrescence is commouly a small soft fungous growth, situated at, or near the verge of the anus. This disease has sometimes been confounded with the hæmorrhoidal tumour, but the two diseases differ completely in structure, and mode of production; and require very different methods of treatment.

236. The hæmorrhoidal excrescence has by some writers been referred, in every instance, to a venereal origin, and it certainly does most frequently spring from this cause; but it occasionally takes place, as I have myself seen, in those who never had a venereal complaint; and Wiseman says he has met with it in an infant.

237. Persons of a relaxed constitution, who with much exercise perspire freely may be considered to be in circumstances favouring the production of this complaint, unless extremely attentive to cleanliness. In one instance, I have known the acrid fumes of burning sulphur bring

on an affection of the skin, terminating in this disease.*

238. When this disease is produced from a venereal cause, it appears to be mostly connected with gonorrhœa, and I believe is generally brought on by this alone; from the purulent matter by means of the linen coming in contact with the verge of the anus, which in this way may excite a similar discharge from the mucous membrane lining the sphincter, acquiring a peculiar acrimony, and eventually inducing that unhealthy state of the cutis round the verge of the anus which generates the excrescence. In these cases the disease is on examination found to excrete a fœtid ichorous discharge, excessive in quantity, and extremely offensive in quality.

Sect. 2.

On the Symptoms and Appearances.

239 Hæmorrhoidal excrescences are generally numerous, very rarely single. They usually make their appearance near the margin or verge of the anus; and generally arise from the inner membrane of the sphincter. Wiseman, to whose extreme diligence and candour the Profession are greatly indebted for much practical observation in surgery, relates a case of this kind in which so many excrescences had formed, as to

* Case 51.

render it difficult to find their insertion. Five of the largest exceeded the length of an inch and a half, and were attached by narrow peduncles to the integuments; while some were found springing from the inner membrane of the gut, fairly beyond the sphincter.

240. M. LIEUTAUD observes, that in examinations after death, they have been found attached to the internal membrane of the rectum, in such number, as to have hindered the passage of the contents of the bowels.

241. Hæmorrhoidal excrescences are either of a bright or a dull red, or lurid colour, of a fungous consistence, easily broken, and readily made to bleed. This is as I have found them, but M. SWEDIAUR observes they are sometimes hard and firm; and they have been described by Mr. B. BELL as occasionally acquiring the consistence of the firmest scirrhus. The last-mentioned gentleman observes, that " these excrescences seem all to be productions of the cuticle;" but, as far as observation and experience have hitherto enabled me to judge, they appear in every instance to originate in disease of the cutis, and not the cuticle.

242. M. DELPECH, who has taken a comprehensive, and, in most particulars, a very correct view of the present state of surgery, observes upon the hæmorrhoidal tumour, " ce que l'on designe par le terme commun d'hæmorrhoides, consiste le plus souvent dans une alteration analogue a ce que nous decrirons ailleurs sous le nom de fungus hæmatodes;" and from the description, as well as treatment recommended, it appears that the tumour and the excrescence

are considered to be only two varieties of one and the same disease; which was precisely the opinion of AMBROSE PARE, in the year 1579.

243. It is certainly true that both these forms of disease may occur in the same patient, but this circumstance alone is no proof of their identity. The hæmorrhoidal tumour is seated in the cellular membrane beneath the skin; the excrescence in the skin itself, or the mucous membrane contiguous with it. The hæmorrhoidal tumour is formed by a deposit of blood, either in dilated veins or cells; the excrescence, on the contrary, is a fungous growth, the vessels of which I believe in no instance enlarge, or pour out their blood into cells.

244. M. LIEUTAUD, speaking of the hæmorrhoidal excrescence, was aware of the importance of the distinction, for he says, " Ces tubercules, qu'on doit bien distinguer des hæmorrhoides fletries, occupent les bords de l'anus." The truth is, that both the disease, and the treatment involve considerations of much higher importance in the one case, than in the other.

245. The hæmorrhoidal excrescence is occasionally connected with the appearance of cracks or fissures, proceeding outwards from the sphincter, in the natural plaits or folds of the skin. These fissures, usually attended with an offensive discharge, so exactly resemble the rhagades that occur in venereal disease, that they have very properly been regarded as a decisive mark of venereal taint in the constitution.

Sect. 3.

On the Treatment.

246. The treatment required will be either local or constitutional. As a local disease, hæmorrhoidal excrescence may be readily cured in almost every instance. Where the excrescences are numerous, and mostly small, they may conveniently enough be removed, by snipping them off with a pair of sharp scissars. In some cases the scalpel may be preferred, where the basis is broad, or extensive. Should the excrescence be single or the patient averse to the knife, a single ligature may be applied round the base of the part to be removed; or if the base is broad, a double ligature upon a curved needle passed through the centre, may be tied on each side.

247. From the structure of the disease, it is obvious that bleeding can never claim attention in whatever manner the removal of the excrescence may be effected. Upon the adoption of excision a little lint constantly wetted with some cold lotion may be laid upon the parts for a few days; they will thus be kept cool until the skin heals over. When the ligature is applied, fomentations may be useful should much pain follow the operation.

248. Where the excrescences are connected not only with a discharge, but with cracks and fissures of the skin, the application of some of the various sedative or astringent solutions, containing either acetate of lead, or the sulphates of copper, zinc or iron, may be directed. Should these fail, alterative medicines may be tried. I have never met with a case where this disease has required the full effect of mercurial excitement in the system for its cure, but it is reasonable to suppose the case may occur, and it will then be necessary to subject the patient to precisely the same means and management adopted for the eradication of any other direct venereal symptom.

CHAPTER VIII.

ON THE MEANS BEST CALCULATED TO ESTABLISH A REGULAR STATE AND ACTION OF THE BOWELS, AS ESSENTIALLY CONDUCIVE TO THE PREVENTION OF MOST OF THE ABOVE DISEASES.

249. OF the numerous diseases to which the human frame is subject, there are but few, very few, that may not either be produced, or greatly aggravated, by habitual derangement in the functions of the alimentary canal. The accustomed usages of society; the nature and quantity of the food we eat; the modes of exercise and of rest, together with our manner of clothing; all appear to me calculated to interfere, more or less, with the regularity of action, and consequently with the proper functions of the bowels. Upon these considerations, however, I confess myself to enter with some degree of diffidence, after having read the comprehensive, and beautifully eloquent papers of Mr. ABERNETHY upon this subject.

250. The original intention of the great Author of nature may be partially traced, in the diversity of provisions appointed for enabling the animal

machine to support itself under the various circumstances in which it may be placed. The different systems of parts of which the body is made up, and the different functions assigned to those systems, display, on many occasions, the most admirable facility, as well as power, of harmonizing with each other, for the promotion of the general good, and the maintenance of health; no one proceeding independently, but each moving forward in unison with the rest. To point out, in illustration of the present remarks, the manner in which any accidental check to perspiration is compensated by an increase in the quantity of fluid separated by the kidnies; to observe how these glands will almost suspend their action when too large a proportion of fluid matter is passing off by the bowels in diarrhœa; or to advert to the temporary influence acknowledged by all the internal secreting organs under any material excess in perspiration, would be a superfluous task. As facts, these circumstances, and many others of a similar nature, are sufficiently familiar; they lead us at least to perceive that the general balance, for the regulation of which so many points have been wisely adjusted, is requisite and necessary for the general good of the economy.

251. The sedentary occupations unavoidably followed by multitudes in civilized life are unfavourable to health, and to the general diffusion of healthy action. The vigour of circulation fails, every impression from external cold is more sensibly felt, suggesting a necessity for warmer clothing; and the habit of clothing the

body too warmly is not unfrequently the means of permanently destroying the balance that ought to subsist between the bowels and the skin. Many persons have an extreme aversion to active exercise, although almost every one must have observed that a brisk walk on a cool day, provided the clothing is not quite impervious, is conducive not only to refreshment, but to the natural action of the bowels. The best proof that we generally sleep much warmer than is proper, is, I think, afforded by those who, from some accident, have been confined for a time to their bed; they all leave it in a comparatively reduced and exhausted condition.

252. As to food, Mr. ABERNETHY very justly remarks, that the ease with which it is obtained is one means of our swallowing much more than is necessary; and, as if excess in quantity was not sufficient, the very mode of its preparation is often such as to create heat, rather than promote digestion.

253. These, and many other circumstances, have a tendency to establish the habit of confinement in the bowels: and, as the known duty of the intestinal tube is that of transmitting its contents, and rejecting that which is no longer useful for the purposes of nutrition, it is natural to conclude that where activity is deficient, it requires to be excited; and upon this ground, stimulating or purgative medicines have been administered.

254. Purgative medicines, then, have the effect of exciting the bowels to action, inducing them

to pass forward their contents. Medicines of this description have also the power of exciting, more or less considerably, an increase in the quantity of fluids poured into the intestinal canal.

255. There is yet another object to be regarded in the exhibition of purgative medicines, an object which is at least equal, or perhaps superior in importance to the rest; it is that of clearing the bowels, not from the refuse of the food, but from certain unhealthy matters the result of morbid secretion, proceeding either from the internal surface of the intestines or from some of the viscera, immediately connected with them. The occasional existence of such matters has been adverted to by the earliest writers; but Mr. ABERNETHY is the first author who has placed them in a clear point of view, and given them their proper consequence, attributing to them, in many cases, an almost absolute influence in producing diseased structure, as well as disturbed function; although in a few instances, perhaps, the secret operation of this powerful cause of disorder has been somewhat overrated.

256. A circumstance that occurred in the year 1808, while doing duty as Surgeon to the 82d Regiment, led me to believe, that in many cases of confinement of bowels, medicines may be so directed as to render purgatives unnecessary.

It happened that an elderly lady, residing at Scarborough, desired my opinion, requesting me to point out, if I could, some plan, by the adoption of which she might obtain a more regular action of her bowels. She had no complaint to make as to her general health; her appetite was good, and she slept well, neither did there appear to be any material defect in the condition of the digestive organs; the only objectionable circumstance being that of her scarcely ever passing a stool without the assistance of medicine. The advice, she said, she had always received from her professional friends was, that when confined in her bowels, she should still have recourse to opening medicines; she added, that really she had taken so great a variety, and so large a quantity, that she loathed the very idea of going on, and felt extremely anxious to know if any plan could be suggested to render it unnecessary.

257. On reflection it appeared probable that this was an instance of deficient action from defective strength, and that, perhaps, by persevering for a time in the use of medicines calculated to restore tone, the bowels might recover the disposition, as well as the power, to propel their contents with regularity; at any rate, it appeared to me there could be no harm in making the experiment. I therefore first ordered the decoction and tincture of bark to be taken daily. This, in a week, appeared to have done neither good nor harm; there was no heat of tongue or skin; but there had been occasion for castor-oil. Decoction of bark was next directed by itself; and in three weeks she thought her inside felt stronger, with less disposition to flatulence than before. In consequence of this amendment

the medicine was continued for a month longer, within which period she found there was no longer any occasion to solicit the action of the bowels at all, a regular and easy motion of occurring every day. This restoration in the tone and action of the bowels appeared likely to be lasting; for there had been no return of the complaint a year and a half afterwards.

258. The adoption of a similar principle, with some slight modifications, has, in a variety of instances, enabled me to restore to the bowels the power of acting from their own impulse, without the perpetual necessity for being reminded of their duty. To set down particular instances would, I apprehend, be loss of time; neither have I preserved accurate notes but of very few. Some of the cases in which this treatment completely succeeded have been mentioned.* I might enumerate many others, the results of which were equally satisfactory. For the present, however, it will be sufficient to observe, that I have, in some instances, at first combined the decoction of bark with a fourth part the quantity of infusion of senna, or with that proportion which answered the purpose of regulating the bowels, occasionally diminishing the quantity of the aperient, till the action of the bowels was observed to go on well with the bark alone.

259. Under some circumstances, the decoction and tincture of bark will answer extremely well together; but the decoction alone is in general, less apt to require a temporary combination

* Case 39. 48. 55, &c.

with Epsom salt, infusion of sinna, or some other aperient.

560. If the innumerable train of ill consequences known to be induced by habitual confinement of bowels are adverted to, there will be no need to excuse the bringing forward any proposition that has for its object the prevention or removal of so great an evil; more particularly while we continue to retain that sort of instinctive feeling which leads us to perfer food to physic.

I am not unconscious that we are all subject to feel the basis of attachment to our own opinions, for which reason the present remarks are brought forward rather as suggestions than as established truths, the practical value of which can only be absolutely determined by their being submitted to the test of more extensive experience. The ability of an individual is almost entirely confined to the power of stating faithfully what he may have watched attentively, within the comparatively narrow circle of his own personal observation.

INDEX.

	Page
ABERNETHY, Mr., his remarks on digestion,	228
Abscess, abdominal, mode of ascertaining,	83
—— in no, causes of danger from,	208
——————, remote consequences of,	209
——————, treatment of,	208
——————, when to be opened,	209
———, from strictured rectum,	11
Accidents may sometimes be made useful,	18
Acrimony to be avoided, in ulcerated bowels,	93
Adhesion, how conducive to safety,	82
————, ill consequences of,	19
————, in the rectum, management of,	18
————, sometimes the means of saving life,	82
Air, change of, sometimes essentially useful,	213
Arteries, exhalent, hæmorrhage from,	85
Astringents, not always successful in hæmorrhage,	97
Bell, Mr. Benj, his account of hæmorrhoidal excrescence,	224
Bladder, diseased, sometimes a cause of prolapsus,	129
Bleeding, in inflammation,	17
————, from within the anus,	175
————————————, treatment of,	177
Blood, enormous quantity vomitted,	83
———, voided per anum, no proof of ulceration,	84
Bodkin extracted from the bladder,	7
Bone sometimes injured by abscess in ano,	208
Bougie, when applicable in strictured rectum,	27
————, improper,	28
Bowels, curious periodical affection of,	22
———, habitual laxity of,	78
———, irritable, importance of,	ib.
———, regular action of, mode of procuring,	228
———————————, necessity for,	178
———, secondary affections of,	83
———, ulcerated, appearance on dissection,	88

INDEX.

	Page
Bowels, ulcerated, favourable progress of,	83
————, peculiarities, when healed,	89
————, ulcer in, sometimes unimportant,	85
Bowman, Mr., his case of intus-susception,	147
Burrel, Dr., his case of stricture,	12
Causes of ulceration in the mucous membrane,	76
Caution, in regard to bleeding,	92
————, necessity for, in delivering an opinion,	93
Cholera morbus, a cause of inflammation,	2
———————————— prolapsus,	128
Colica pictonum, a cause of prolapsus,	129
Collins, Mr., his case of tympany,	21
Colon, stricture in,	12
Contraction, in the rectum, sometimes escapes detection,	30
Costiveness, a frequent cause of piles,	169
Delpech, M., case of tumours in the rectum,	120
————, opinion on hæmorrhoidal tumours,	225
————, opinions upon stricture,	14
————, treatment of scirrhous stricture,	32
Deranged bowels, importance of,	78
Desault, M., case of tumour operated upon,	126
————, opinion on tumours in the rectum,	119
————, practice in stricture,	30
————, remarks on stricture,	14
Diet to be carefully regulated in ulcerated bowels,	93
Diseases, internal, negligent treatment of,	16
Dysentery, a cause of prolapsus	128
Effused lymph, great strength acquired by,	19
Effusion, from inflammation, consequences of,	8
Enema, useful by volume as well as warmth,	90
Eruptions, repelled, a cause of stricture,	3
Excrescence, hæmorrhoidal,	222
Extraneous bodies, in the rectum, effects of,	3
Fæcal matters retained, occasional consequences of,	24
Fatal constipation, from a sacculus in the bowels,	25
Fish-bones, consequence of swallowing,	26
————, mode of removing from the rectum,	ib.
Fistula, appearance of, on dissection,	207
————, causes of,	203
————, consequences of neglecting,	205
————, importance of, dependant on habit,	ib.
————, mode of operating for,	211
————, nature of,	204

INDEX.

	Page
Fistula, symptoms of,	204
———, treatment of,	208
Fruit-stones, consequences of swallowing,	22
Fume of tobacco, unskilfully used, may prove fatal,	145
Gangrenous state of the bowels,	79
Hæmorrhage, after operating, how restrained,	213
————, capillary, treatment of,	97
————, returns of effects on the system,	172
Haemorrhoidal bleeding, conditions under which it occurs,	176
———————— *diseases*, reflections on the consequences of,	180
———————— *excrescence*, causes of,	222
————————————, generally of venereal origin,	223
————————————, symptoms of,	225
————————————, treatment of,	226
———————— *tumour*, bleeding from,	171
————————, causes of,	169
————————, mode of production,	170
————————, often the effect of a ruptured vessel,	173
————————, operation for the removal of,	178
————————, sanguineous and serous,	170
————————, structure of,	173
————————, symptoms of,	160
————————, treatment of,	176
Heat, internal, a symptom of inflamed rectum,	5
Heaviside, Mr., cured prolapsus by the ligature,	139
————————, his remarks on spontaneous mortification	173
————————, treatment of obstinate costiveness	20
Hey, Mr, case of tumour in the rectum,	118
————, mode of treating prolapsus,	139
Hill, Mr., case of diseased and mortified rectum,	83
————, case of stricture,	12
Hog's bristles, stricture produced by,	13
Holmes, Dr., his case of stricture,	13
Home, Sir Everard, his work on stricture,	17
Hooper, Dr., his morbid anatomical collection,	13
————————, specimen of tumour in the bowel,	121
————————, treatment in cases of ulceration,	94
Huxham, Dr., history of diseased bowels,	79
Inflamed rectum, state of,	9
Inflammation, a cause of stricture,	1
——————, effects of, in the weak and irritable,	6
——————, effusion from,	6
——————, erysipelatous, treatment of,	210
——————, gangrenous,	210

INDEX.

	Page
Inflammation, occasional difficulty in discerning,	20
———, poritoneal, how produced,	81
———, unhealthy, in abscess,	205
Internal diseases, negligent treatment of,	16
Intus-susception, explained,	133
———, may appear outwardly as a prolapsus,	135
———, mode of distinguishing,	ib.
———, most fatal in children,	134
———, requires promptitude and ability,	144
Irritability, extreme, allied to the scorbutic diathesis,	78
Irritable bladder, a consequence of abscess near it,	206
———, treatment of,	210
Irritation, a cause of ulceration,	77
———, in the rectum, treatment of,	211
Johnson, Dr., remarks on atmospheric influence,	77
Judgment required in applying the ligature,	141
Lieutaud, M., observations on prolapsus,	132
———, remarks on hæmorrhoidal excrescence,	224
Ligature, application of, to tumour in the rectum,	125
———, mode of applying, for prolapsus,	140
———, rarely productive of inconvenience,	179
Liver and skin, sympathy between,	77
Lumbal muscles, spasm of, from loaded bowels,	25
Lymph effused, a consequence of inflammation,	2
Management, after recovery from ulceration,	98
Malaena, interesting case of,	87
Membranous bands, in the rectum,	9
Objects, to be regarded, in using the bougie,	28
Obstinate costiveness, a sign of intus-susception,	141
Odier, Professor, curious observation by,	24
Operating, improper in certain states of habit,	213
Operation, for fistula, mode of performed,	211
———, — hæmorrhoidal tumours,	178
———, — prolapsus ani,	139
Operations require subsequent attention,	3
Opium, its excellent effects in stricture,	32
Parents, caution to,	141
Peritoneal inflammation, how induced by ulceration,	81
Piles, or hæmorrhoidal tumours, causes of,	169
———, inflamed, extreme pain from,	171
Plum-stones, fatal consequences from swallowing,	22
Portal, M., memoir upon internal bleeding,	86

INDEX.

	Page
Pott, Mr, opinions upon fistula in ano,	206
Prolapsed bowel, change in, from exposure to air,	132
Prolapsus ani, causes of,	128
—————, inflamed and constricted, treatment of,	139
—————, mode of reducing,	137
—————, the consequence of relaxation,	131
—————, treatment of,	136
—————, quantity sometimes very large,	130
Purulent matter, in the stools, argues ulceration,	125
Reasons for leaving a tumour when tied,	126
Rectum, inflammation of, may suspend labour,	5
———————, may produce retention of urine,	ib.
Relaxation of bowels, importance of,	91
————— the structure of the bowel demonstrated to exist in prolapsus,	131
Renton, Mr., valuable case of intus-susception,	147
Rodamel, M,, excellent case of bleeding from the bowels,	87
Sinus; nature and cause of,	204
Sloane Dr., consequence of eating strawberries, related by,	24
Sloughing, of varicose veins;	133
Spasm, intestinal, removed by mechanical irritation,	87
Spasmodic disorder of bowels, curious instance of,	23
Sphincter, spasm of, treatment of,	177
Stoker, Dr., case of diseased bowels,	82
Stools, appearance of blood in,	84
Strangulation, an occasional consequence of prolapsus,	133
Stricture, in the rectum, causes of,	1
—————, from spasm of the sphincter,	4
—————, high up in the bowel,	12
—————, occurs spontaneously,	3
—————, scirrhous,	4
—————, appearances in,	14
—————, characters of,	12
—————, symptoms of,	5
—————, treatment of,	16
—————, urgent straining, a consequence of,	10
Tenesmus, a sign of inflamed rectum,	5
Tobacco fume, use of, in intus-susception,	143
—————, mode of applying,	144
————— its operation,	145
Tumour, hæmorrhoidal, operation for,	178
——, in the rectum, causes of,	118
—————, hæmorrhage from,	124
—————, removal of, by ligature,	125

INDEX.

	Page
Tumour in the rectum, structure of,	122
———————————, treatment of,	123
———————————, ulcerated, treatment of,	125
Ulcer, in the bowels, may result from a bruise,	80
———, in the rectum, local treatment of,	95
Ulcerated bowels, the effect of combined causes,	80
————— surface when healed, peculiarities of,	89
————— tumour of, uncertain event,	125
Ulceration, a consequence of stricture,	9
—————, circumscribed or diffused,	81
—————, how produced,	6
—————; in stricture, occasionl effect of,	15
—————, of the mucous membrane of the bowel,	76
—————, symptoms of,	80
—————, treatment of,	90
Veins, varicose, between the coats of the rectum,	176
———, sloughing of, in prolapsus,	133
Venereal disease, a supposed cause of stricture,	2
Warm-bath, trial of its power,	91
Wiseman, his account of the hæmorrhoidal excrescence,	223
Yonge, Mr., curious case related by,	22

THE END.

SD - #0042 - 141022 - C0 - 229/152/14 - PB - 9780260238672 - Gloss Lamination